Evaluation of Continuing Education in the Health Professions

Evaluation in Education and Human Services

Editors:

George F. Madaus, Boston College, Chestnut
  Hill, Massachusetts, U.S.A.
Daniel L. Stufflebeam, Western Michigan
  University, Kalamazoo, Michigan, U.S.A.

Previously published books in the series:

Evaluation of Continuing Education in the Health Professions

edited by

Stephen Abrahamson
University of Southern
California School of Medicine

Based on a Conference presented by
The University of Southern California
Development and Demonstration Center in
Continuing Education for Health Professionals
(A project of the W.K. Kellogg Foundation)

Kluwer · Nijhoff Publishing
a member of the Kluwer Academic Publishers Group
Boston   Dordrecht   Lancaster

Distributors for North America:
Kluwer Academic Publishers
190 Old Derby Street
Hingham, MA 02043, U.S.A.

Distributors for all other countries:
Kluwer Academic Publishers Group
Distribution Centre
P.O. Box 322
3300AH Dordrecht,
The Netherlands

Library of Congress Cataloging in Publication Data
Main entry under title:

Evaluation of continuing education in the health professions.

(Evaluation in education and human services)
"Based on a conference presented by the Development and
Demonstration Center in Continuing Education for Health
Professionals (a project of the W.K. Kellogg Foundation)."
Includes index.
1. Medicine — Study and teaching (Continuing education) —
Evaluation — Congresses. 2. Medical education — Evaluation —
Congresses. I. Abrahamson, Stephen. II. University of Southern
California. Development and Demonstration Center in Continuing
Education for Health Professionals. III. W.K. Kellogg Foundation.
IV. Series. [DNLM: 1. Education, Medical, Continuing —
congresses. 2. Evaluation Studies — congresses. W 20 E92]
R845.E9   1985   610'.7'15   85-2286
ISBN 0-89838-168-1

Printed in the United States of America

Contents

Contributing Authors

Stephen Abrahamson, Ph.D., Director, Division of Research in Medical Education and Professor (Chairman), Department of Medical Education, University of Southern California School of Medicine

Deborah Burkett, Ed.D., Formerly Research Assistant, Development and Demonstration Center in Continuing Education for Health Professionals, University of Southern California

William W. Cooley, Ed.D., Director of Evaluation Research at the Learning Research and Development Center and Professor of Education at the University of Pittsburgh

Teri Denson, Ph.D., Formerly Director of Evaluation, Development and Demonstration Center in Continuing Education for Health Professionals, University of Southern California

Joseph S. Green, Ph.D., Formerly Deputy Director, Development and Demonstration Center in Continuing Education for Health Professionals, University of Southern California and currently Associate Director of the Southwest Regional Medical Education Center, Long Beach Veterans Administration

Kaaren I. Hoffman, Ph.D., Associate Professor of Medical Education, University of Southern California School of Medicine

George F. Madaus, D.Ed., Director of the Center for the Study of Testing, Evaluation and Educational Policy, Boston College

Phil R. Manning, M.D., Director of the Development and Demonstration Center in Continuing Education for Health Professionals and Associate Vice President for Continuing Education in the Health Professions, University of Southern California, and the Paul Ingalls Hoagland Professor of Continuing Medical Education.

James T. Martinoff, Ph.D., Director of Curriculum Development, School of Pharmacy, and Associate Clinical Professor of Medical Education, School of Medicine, University of Southern California

Julie G. Nyquist, Ph.D., Assistant Professor of Clinical Medical Education, University of Southern California

Daniel L. Stufflebeam, Ph.D., Director of the Evaluation Center and Professor, Faculty of Educational Leadership, Western Michigan University

Richard M. Wolf, Ph.D., Professor of Psychology and Education, Teachers College, Columbia University

Foreword
Phil R. Manning

"Can you prove that continuing education really makes any difference?" Over the years, educators concerned with continuing education (CE) for health professionals have either heard or voiced that question in one form or another more than once. But because of the difficulty in measuring the specific effects of a given course, program, or conference, the question has not been answered satisfactorily. Since CE is costly, since CE is now mandated in some states for re-registration, and since its worth has not been proven in formal evaluation research, the pressure to evaluate remains strong.

The question can be partially answered by a more careful definition of continuing education, particularly the goals to be achieved by CE. Another part of the answer depends on the development of a stronger commitment to evaluation of CE by its providers. But a significant part of the answer might be provided through the improvement of methods used in evaluation of continuing education for health professionals.

To address this last concern, the Development and Demonstration Center in Continuing Education for the Health Professions of the University of Southern California organized and conducted a meeting of academicians and practitioners in evaluation of continuing education. During a three-day period, participants heard formal presentations by five invited speakers and then discussed the application of the state of the art of educational evaluation to problems of evaluation of continuing education for health professionals.

The original idea for the Conference came from the National Institutes of Health Consensus Development Conferences in which recognized experts in a given area of health care gather and arrive at consensus with regard to management of a given medical problem. Our view was that there were experts in educational evaluation with little or no experience in continuing education for health professionals who might be asked to reach consensus on optimum approaches to evaluation of CE. Such a small-but-elite gathering might help resolve major questions besetting CE evaluators, such as whether to rely upon "pure" experimental design or instead use the "naturalistic" study approach.

As the planning sessions evolved, however, it became clear that such "consensus" was beyond the state of the art or was even contraindicated by the diversity of CE activities. Thus the planners, instead, decided to use a panel of nationally recognized experts in educational evaluation with little or no experience in continuing education for health professionals to present the state of the art of different aspects of evaluation and then to involve the conference participants in discussion of those principles applicable to real problems of continuing education for health professionals.

This book includes the presentations by the five experts in educational evaluation. It also includes chapters prepared by evaluators of the Center and faculty members of the Department of Medical Education of the University of Southern California. These special chapters include both summaries of participant reactions to the expert presentations and additional views on those specific areas of evaluation. Thus the book juxtaposes basic principles of educational evaluation and their application to real problems of evaluation of continuing education for health professionals.

In addition, this book reflects on some of the basic questions that kept recurring during the three days. To what extent must the evaluator decide what is to be evaluated? Should evaluation be limited to knowledge gain in clinical subjects? Is evaluation synonymous with experimental research? To what extent must evaluation be concerned with physician practices? Is patient outcome to be considered the only valid measure of the success of continuing education for health professionals?

The methods of traditional continuing education have not changed for decades. Physicians still continue their education by reading journals and books, attending courses and conferences, and informally discussing medical problems with colleagues. There are many anecdotes indicating that these methods have been successful in changing the physician's performance. Physicians use innovations such as ultrasound and computed axial tomography, newer drugs such as the calcium channel blockers, and learn about "new diseases" such as Legionnaires' Disease, toxic shock, and AIDS, even though they completed formal training before the new developments were described. Pre- and post-course testing shows that physicians do learn facts by attending courses and conferences. Thus traditional continuing education provides a mechanism of information transfer that gives the physician a framework upon which to build an understanding of the state of the art. It is unrealistic to expect continuing medical education to provide many answers to specific problems in practice. Practice-centered study through consulting journals, books, and colleagues on specific issues is necessary. Thus part of the difficulty with evaluation of general unfocused continuing education is that we are trying to document outcomes that can not be expected. Does this mean that there is no need to evaluate continuing medical education? Emphatically not!

Indeed, there is more of a need than ever before. With the increase in the cost of continuing education (cost that must be paid by the health professional only to be passed on to the consumer and thus add to the already criticized cost of health care), providers of continuing education have an obligation to evaluate their programs no matter what the form and no matter what the goals. Continuing education providers cannot be content with head-counting data or happiness indexes. Now is the time to harness the power of the latest in evaluation techniques and put it to work in our arena.

The book takes a significant step in this direction. Basic standards of educational evaluation are discussed; problems in evaluation design, data collection, and data analysis are reviewed; political issues are aired. For those concerned with continuing education for health professionals and its evaluation, this book should prove interesting and informative.

Evaluation of Continuing Education in the Health Professions

1 THE NEED, THE CONFERENCE, THE BOOK

Joseph S. Green

A generally recognized purpose of continuing education (CE) in the health professions is to impact on health practitioners' knowledge and attitudes, their skills in providing health care, and on health-care outcomes of patients (Green et al., 1984). An important purpose of evaluation efforts in CE is to demonstrate the causal links between a given educational activity and one of the aforementioned desirable outcome measures (Abrahamson, 1968). The purpose of this book is to summarize the proceedings of a conference held in 1983 to study the "State of the Art of Evaluation of Continuing Education Activities in the Health Professions." This chapter outlines the need for such a gathering, describes the faculty, participants, and format for the evaluation dialogue, and orients the reader to the format and purpose of the remainder of the book.

The Need

In 1979 the University of Southern California (USC) School of Medicine, with assistance from the W.K. Kellogg Foundation, established the Development and Demonstration Center in Continuing Education for Health

1

Professionals for the express purpose of examining the most effective and efficient methods of CE. In order to accomplish this goal, an in-depth study of CE evaluation was initiated. Partially on the basis of a study undertaken by Lloyd and Abrahamson (1979) entitled "Effectiveness of Continuing Medical Education: A Review of the Evidence," the idea developed for a consensus-type conference to initiate a dialogue between nationally known experts in educational evaluation theory and methodology and CE evaluation practitioners. The idea was simple: establish a forum for bringing the expertise of educational researchers to bear on the real-world problems of those involved in evaluation CE in the health professions.

The efficiency of continuing education in medicine, as well as the other health professions, has long been called into question by a number of critics (Storey, 1978; Brown and Uhl, 1970; Miller, 1967; Bertram and Brooks-Bertram, 1977). Four specific arguments continually surface: (1) CE activities are rarely designed to bring about changes in the competence or performance of health professionals (Walsh, 1981); (2) even if they are systematically developed, the evaluation design most often does not lead to definitive judgments about the impact of the educational endeavors (Green and Walsh, 1979); (3) the principles of rigorous scientific inquiry and controlled experimentation are impractical in the unstructured reality of CE in the health professions; and, (4) the measurement of health professionals' competence and performance (let alone health-care outcomes) has not developed to the point where baseline and subsequent change measures are obtainable (Williamson et al., 1967).

The Conference

In 1982 the Development and Demonstration Center in Continuing Education for Health Professionals in collaboration with the Division of Research in Medical Education within the USC School of Medicine put together a planning committee (see figure 1-1) to develop a conference to study the state of the art of educational evaluation to determine the implications for CE evaluation.

The Conference was designed after a careful analysis of problems that were discussed in the CE evaluation literature and from information that emerged from a survey of the medical education evaluators at USC School of Medicine (n = 15). That survey uncovered several high-priority CE evaluation problems.

- How can the evaluator best achieve the appropriate match between the data-analysis techniques and the quality of the data collected?

UNIVERSITY OF SOUTHERN CALIFORNIA
DEVELOPMENT AND DEMONSTRATION CENTER
IN CONTINUING EDUCATION FOR HEALTH PROFESSIONALS
A Project of the W.K. Kellogg Foundation

presents a conference on

EVALUATION OF CONTINUING EDUCATION
IN THE HEALTH PROFESSIONS:

THE STATE OF THE ART

February 4-6, 1983

Huntington Sheraton Hotel   Pasadena, California

Conference Planning Committee

Stephen Abrahamson, Ph.D., Director, Division of Research in Medical Education, USC School of Medicine

Deborah Burkett, M.A., Research Associate, USC Development and Demonstration Center, Conference Coordinator

Teri A. Denson, Ph.D., Senior Evaluator, USC Development and Demonstration Center, Conference Co-Chairman

Joseph S. Green, Ph.D., Deputy Director, USC Development and Demonstration Center, Conference Co-Chairman

Phil R. Manning, M.D., USC Associate Vice President of Health Affairs, and Director, USC Development and Demonstration Center

Julie Gayle Nyquist, Ph.D., Assistant Professor, Clinical Medical Education, USC School of Medicine

Daniel L. Stufflebeam, Ph.D., Director of the Evaluation Center, and Professor, Faculty of Educational Leadership at Western Michigan University

Figure 1-1. Conference Planning Committee

- Who should make the decisions concerning the evaluation-study design?
- How do we solve the tradeoff involved in using "invasive" data-collection techniques providing "hard" data and noninvasive techniques yielding "soft" data?
- How can qualitative data and quantitative data best be "merged"?
- Is rigid experimental design possible or desirable when what is to be evaluated is real-world CE activities?

The format of the Conference (see figure 1–2) that emerged was one that would allow experts to speak about the state of the art in one of five aspects of evaluation:

1. standards for CE evaluation;
2. design problems;
3. data-collection problems;
4. data-analysis problems;
5. politics of evaluation.

The following were the faculty who were selected to discuss these specifics of evaluation.

Standards:

Daniel L. Stufflebeam, Ph.D., is the Director of the Evaluation Center and Professor, Faculty of Educational Leadership at Western Michigan University. He has 16 years of research and development experience which includes development of approximately 100 standardized achievement tests, several evaluation systems, and the CIPP Evaluation Model; investigation of the item-sampling technique; and study of the 1977 energy crisis, Columbus, Ohio, and its effects on Columbus Public Schools. Dr. Stufflebeam was Chair of the Joint Committee on Standards for the Evaluation of Educational Programs, Projects and Materials.

Design:

Richard M. Wolf, Ph.D., is Professor of Psychology and Education at Teachers College Columbia, New York. He was formerly Assistant Professor of Education at the University of Southern California, Research Associate at the University of Chicago, and Specialist in Education Evaluation, Measurement and Statisics. He is the author of five books and monographs including *Evaluation in Education* and editor (with Ralph Tyler) of *Crucial Issues in Testing*. Dr. Wolf is a consultant to various educational institutions, health-care agencies, governments, and businesses on matters of evaluation, research, and data analysis both in the United States and abroad.

Data Collection:

George F. Madaus, D.Ed., is the Director of the Center for the Study of Testing, Evaluation, and Educational Policy. He completed his postdoctoral work at the University of Chicago in 1966. He has authored or coauthored seven books including the following: *Sources of Difference in School Achievement*; *Evaluation to Improve Learning*; and *The Effects of Standardized Testing*. He was a member of the Joint Committee on Standards for the Evaluation of Educational Programs, Projects, and Materials. Currently he is a member of a joint committee to revise test standards for APA-AERA-NCME (American Psychological Association-American Educational Research Association-National Council on Measurement in Education).

Data Analysis:

William Cooley, Ed.D., is Professor of Education at the University of Pittsburgh and the Director of Evaluation Research at the Learning Research and Development Center. He was Co-director of the Center from 1969–1977. Prior to joining the faculty of the University of Pittsburgh, he was Director of Project TALENT at the American Institute for Research. During the 1972–73 academic year he was a Fellow at the Center for Advanced Study in the Behavioral Sciences. He was the President of the American Educational Research Association (AERA). His present activities are concerned with designing ways of providing useful evaluation services within school districts.

Politics:

Stephen Abrahamson, Ph.D., is Professor and Chairman of the Department of Medical Education in the School of Medicine, and Professor of Education in the School of Education, University of Southern California. Widely recognized as a pioneer in evaluation of medical education, he has been an invited consultant to more than half of the American medical schools. Internationally known as well, he has been a consultant in numerous projects abroad, sponsored by the World Health Organization. Starting in 1963, the Division of Research in Medical Education, of which he is the Director, has conducted many significant national evaluation studies in medical education.

After each address the participants (see figure 1–3) were assigned to small groups (which were multidisciplinary in nature) in order to discuss their reaction to the state of the art. In order to accomplish this, the groups were given typical problems described in a vignette. Using this vignette, the groups were asked to discuss the relevant standards from the *Joint Committee on Standards for Educational Evaluation: Standards for Evaluations of Educational Programs, Projects, and Materials*. They were also asked to react to how the state of the art might suggest new approaches or, on the other hand, how what was presented was impractical. This same format was followed

DAY ONE, Friday, February 4, 1983

Wentworth Room

1:30 to 2:00	Registration
2:00 to 2:30	Welcome by Phil R. Manning, M.D. Overview of conference and introduction of speakers — Joseph S. Green, Ph.D., Moderator
2:30 to 3:15	Keynote Address — "Application of the Joint Committee *Standards* to Evaluation of CE in the Health Professions" — Daniel Stufflebeam, Ph.D.

Ship Room

3:30 to 4:45	Small Group Session #1 Discussion of Heartmobile Proposal in relation to Dr. Stufflebeam's presentation and the *Standards*

Wentworth Room

4:45 to 5:15	Large Group Recap and Summary: Reaction Panel Small group leaders Teri Denson, Ph.D., Chair
5:15 to 6:15	Host Bar Conversation hour with speakers

DAY TWO, Saturday, February 5, 1983

Wentworth Room

9:00 to 9:15	Outline of Day's Activities — Moderator
9:15 to 10:00	Presentation — Design Problems in Evaluation — Richard M. Wolf, Ph.D.

Ship Room

10:00 to 11:30	Small Group Session #2 Discussion of Design Problems of Heartmobile Proposal in relation to Dr. Wolf's presentation and the *Standards*

Wentworth Room

11:30 to 12:15	Large Group Recap and Summary: Small group leaders — James Martinoff, Ph.D., Chair

Figure 1-2. Conference Schedule

DAY TWO, Saturday, February 5, 19& 3 (continued)

Georgian Room

12:15 to 1:15   Lunch — Buffet Provided

Wentworth Room

 1:15 to 2:00   Presentation — Data Collection Problems in Evalua-
                       tion — George F. Madaus, Ed.D.

Ship Room

 2:00 to 3:30   Small Group Session #3

                       Discussion of Data Collection Problems in relation to
                       Dr. Madaus' presentation and the *Standards*

Wentworth Room

 3:30 to 4:15   Large Group Recap and Summary:
                       Small group leaders — Julie Nyquist, Ph.D., Chair

 4:15 to 5:00   Reaction Panel — Richard M. Wolf, Ph.D., George F.
                       Madaus, D.Ed., Joseph S. Green, Ph.D., Chair

 5:00   Conference Evaluation — Julie Nyquist, Ph.D.

 5:10   Adjourn

Ship Room

 6:00   Dinner — Buffet Provided

DAY THREE, Sunday, February 6, 1983

Wentworth Room

 9:00 to 9:15   Outline of Day's Activities — Moderator

 9:15 to 10:00   Presentation — Analysis Problems in Evaluation —
                       William Cooley, Ed.D.

Ship Room

10:00 to 11:30   Small Group Session #4

                       Discussion of Analysis Problems in relation to Dr.
                       Cooley's presentation and the *Standards*

Georgian Room

12:15 to 1:15   Lunch — Buffet Provided

Figure 1–2 (continued)

DAY THREE, Sunday, February 6, 1983 (continued)

Wentworth Room

1:15 to 2:00	Presentation — Politics of Evaluation — Stephen Abrahamson, Ph.D.

Ship Room

2:00 to 3:30	Small Group Session #5
	Discussion of Politics of Evaluation in relation to Dr. Abrahamson's presentation and the *Standards*

Wentworth Room

3:30 to 4:15	Large Group Recap Summary: Small group leaders, Teri Denson, Ph.D.
4:15 to 5:00	Reaction Panel — William Cooley, Ed.D., Stephen Abrahamson, Ph.D., Joseph Green, Ph.D., Chair
5:00 to 5:30	Wrap-up Session — Joseph Green, Ph.D., and Daniel Stufflebeam, Ph.D.
5:30	Conference Evaluation — Julie Nyquist, Ph.D.

Mirror Room

5:40	Unwind at No-Host Bar

Figure 1–2 (continued)

after each presentation. In each of the small groups two members of USC evaluation staff served as "recappers" and "scribes" in order to capture the state of affairs as depicted by the evaluation practitioners. Panel discussions followed each presentation and small-group interaction in order to provide further dialogue between experts and practitioners.

The entire Conference consisted of 71 participants including the five faculty members and the USC staff. The majority of evaluators were from continuing medical education; however, there was a good cross-section of evaluators involved in CE in nursing, dentistry, pharmacy, and allied health. Participants represented 16 states, the District of Columbia, and British Columbia; and they were from professional schools, hospitals, universities, professional associations, government, and private enterprise.

The Book

The purpose of this book is to share with the readers the outcomes of this Conference. The chapters that follow will combine two presentations on

EVALUATION OF CONTINUING-EDUCATION ACTIVITIES
IN THE HEALTH PROFESSIONS:
THE STATE OF THE ART

February 4-6, 1983

Huntington Sheraton Hotel   Pasadena, California

ABRAHAMSON, Stephen, Ph.D., Director, Division of Research in Medical Education, USC School of Medicine; 2025 Zonal Avenue, KAM 200, Los Angeles, California 90033; (213)224-7038.

ADAMCIK, Barbara, M.A., Research Associate, USC School of Pharmacy; 2025 Zonal Avenue, KAM 307A, Los Angeles, California 90033; (213)224-7431.

ALTEMUS, Leonard, D.D.S., D.S.C., Howard University College of Dentistry; 3609 Georgia Avenue N.W., Washington, D.C. 20010; (202)636-5450.

BARTENSTEIN, Shelley, M.S., Research Associate, USC School of Medicine; 2025 Zonal Avenue, KAM 200, Los Angeles, California 90033; (213)224-7038.

BASHOOK, Philip, Ed.D., Michael Reese Hospital & Medical Center, School of Health Sciences, EDU, 29th & Ellis Avenue, Chicago, Illinois; (312)791-5530.

BRUNNER, Marjorie L., School of Allied Medical Professions, Ohio State University; 1583 Perry Street, Columbus, Ohio 43210; (514)422-5618.

BURKETT, Deborah, M.A., Conference Coordinator, USC School of Medicine; 2025 Zonal Avenue, Los Angeles, California 90033; (213)224-7465.

CARTWRIGHT, Charles, B.A., D.D.S., University of Michigan, School of Dentistry; 1000 Kellogg, Ann Arbor, Michigan 48105; (313)763-5070.

CAUFFMAN, Joy G., Ph.D., Director of Postgraduate Education Program in Family and Preventive Medicine, USC School of Medicine, San Pablo Street, PMB-B205, Los Angeles, California 90033; (213)224-7495.

CLINTWORTH, William A., M.L.S., Project Director/Information Broker, Norris Medical Library, USC School of Medicine; 2025 Zonal Avenue, Los Angeles, California 90033; (213)224-7388.

COOLEY, William, Ed.D., Professor of Education, University of Pittsburgh, and Director of Evaluation Research at the Learning Research and Development Center; University of Pittsburgh, Pittsburgh, Pennsylvania, 15260; (412)624-4831.

DENSON, Teri A., Ph.D., Senior Evaluator, Development and Demonstration Center, USC School of Medicine; 2025 Zonal Avenue, KAM 314, Los Angeles, California 90033; (213)224-7743.

EAGAN, Pamela, M.S., M.A., Associate Director, Community Pharmacy Enhancement Project; USC School of Pharmacy, 1985 Zonal Avenue, Los Angeles, California 90033; (213)224-7748.

EVANS, Leonard, Ph.D., Associate Clinical Professor, USC School of Medicine; 2025 Zonal Avenue, KAM 200, Los Angeles, California 90033; (213)224-7038.

Figure 1-3. Roster of Conference Participants

FERGUSON, Kristi, Ph.D., Office of Consultation and Research in Medical Education, The University of Iowa, 2351 CH, Iowa City, Iowa 52242; (319)353-6781.

FIELDING, David, Ed.D., University of British Columbia, Faculty School of Pharmacy, Vancouver, B.C. V6T 1W5 Canada; (604)228-3085.

FORSYTH, Roger, M.D., Southern California Kaiser Permanente Medical Group, Los Angeles, California.

GAINES, Elaine, Ph.D., Charles R. Drew Postgraduate Medical School, 2304 West 79th Street, Inglewood, California 90305; (213)603-4965.

GATES, Jerry, Ph.D., Director of Education and Training, International Group, National Medical Enterprises, Inc.; 2901 Twenty-Eighth Street, P.O. Box 2140, Santa Monica, California 90406; (213)952-4444.

GAZZILLI, Albert, DuPont Clinical Systems, 1480 N. Claremont Boulevard, Claremont, California 91711; (714)626-2451, Ext. 418.

GERBERT, Barbara, Ph.D., University of California, San Francisco; 1483 Fourth Avenue, San Francisco, California 94143; (415)666-3000.

GIRARD, Roger A., Ph.D., Assistant Professor of Medical Education, USC School of Medicine; 2025 Zonal Avenue, Los Angeles, California 90033; (213)224-7038.

GREEN, Joseph S., Ph.D., Deputy Director, Development and Demonstration Center, USC School of Medicine, 2025 Zonal Avenue, KAM 300, Los Angeles, California 90033; (213)224-7743.

GROSSWALD, Sarina, Association of American Medical Colleges, Suite 200/ DERP, One Dupont Circle, N.W., Washington, D.C.; (202)828-0650.

HAJEK, Anna Marie, Triton College Continuing Education Center, 2000 Fifth Avenue (CECHP RC208) River Grove, Illinois 60171; (312)456-80005.

HAYASHI, Jo Anne, University of Texas Health Science Center at San Antonio, Office of the Dean, Continuing Dental Education, 7703 Floyd Curl Drive, San Antonio, Texas 78284; (512)691-7451.

HOFFMAN, Kaaren I., Ph.D., Associate Professor of Medical Education, USC School of Medicine; 2025 Zonal Avenue, Los Angeles, California 90033; (213)224-7038.

HOLLEY, Linka, M.S.N., North Central RMEC, 5445 Minnehaha Avenue South, Minneapolis, Minnesota 55417; (612)725-6537.

IVERSON, Patricia, Oregon Health Sciences University, Division of Continuing Medical Education, The Oregon Health Sciences University, Portland, Oregon 95201; (503)225-8700.

JACOBS, Saul, M.A., Sutherland Learning Associates, 8700 Reseda Boulevard, Suite 108, Northridge, California 91324; (213)701-1344.

Figure 1–3 (continued)

KEARNS, Karen, M.S., Research Associate, USC School of Medicine; 2025 Zonal Avenue, Los Angeles, California 90033; (213)224-7038.

KROCHALK, Pamela, Dr.P.H., Evaluation Specialist/Clinical Instructor, USC School of Medicine; 2025 Zonal Avenue, Los Angeles, California; (213)224-7587.

LAWRENCE, Kenneth, M.F.A., Continuing Education Center, V.A. Medical Center, 50 Irving Street, N.W., Washington, D.C. 20412.

LENOSKI, Edward, M.D., Assistant Professor of Emergency Medicine, USC School of Medicine, LAC/USC Medical Center; PDP 2D4, 1200 North State Street, Los Angeles, California 90033; (213)226-3691.

LERNER, Judith, M.Ed., V.A. Southwest Regional Medical Education Center, 5901 East Seventh Street, Long Beach, California 90822; (213)498-6821.

MADAUS, George F., D.Ed., Director of Center for Study of Testing, Evaluation, and Educational Policy, Boston College, Chestnut Hill, Massachusetts 02167; (617)969-0100, Ext. 4521.

MANNING, Phil R., M.D., Associate Dean, Continuing Medical Education; Director, Development & Demonstration Center, USC School of Medicine; 2025 Zonal Ave., KAM 307, Los Angeles, California 90033; (213)224-7047.

MARTIN, Karen, M.S.N., The Visiting Nurse Association of Omaha; 10840 Harney Circle, Omaha, Nebraska 68154; (402)334-1820, Ext. 138.

MARTINOFF, James T., Ph.D., Director of Curriculum Development and Pharmacy Instruction, USC School of Pharmacy; 1985 Zonal Avenue, PSC 700, Los Angeles, California 90033; (213)224-7501.

MCGRAW, Phyllis, M.S., Research Associate, USC School of Medicine; 2025 Zonal Avenue, KAM 200, Los Angeles, California 90033; (213)224-7038.

MEANS, Robert P., Ph.D., Assistant Director of Continuing Education, Office of Postgraduate Medicine and Health Professions Education, Towsley Center, Ann Arbor, Michigan 48109.

MENDENHALL, Robert C., Assistant Clinical Professor of Clinical Medical Education, USC School of Medicine; 2025 Zonal Avenue, KAM 200, Los Angeles, California 90033; (213)224-7038.

MOORE, Willis, Ph.D., Wayne State University, 525 Health Science Building WSU, Detroit, Michigan 58202; (313)577-1714.

MORGAN, Eunice, M.S.N., California State University, Long Beach, Department of Nursing; 1250 Bellflower Boulevard, Long Beach, California 90840; (213)498-4452.

MURCHISON-WARNER, Norma, M.A., Veterans Administration Regional Medical Education Center, 5901 East Seventh Street, Long Beach, California 90822; (213)498-1313, Ext. 3121.

Figure 1-3 (continued)

NEWTON, David S., Ph.D., Auburn University, School of Pharmacy, Auburn, Alabama 36849; (205)826-4037.

NYQUIST, Julie G., Ph.D., Assistant Professor, Clinical Medical Education, USC School of Medicine; 2025 Zonal Avenue, KAM 200, Los Angeles, California 90033; (213)224-7038.

PENNINGTON, Floyd, Ph.D., Arthritis Foundation, 13143 Spring Street N.W., Atlanta, Georgia 30309; (404)872-7100.

POLLACK, Susan, M.S., USC Instructional Services, School of Business, Los Angeles, California 90089-1421; (213)743-1421.

RACE, George J., M.D., Ph.D., Associate Dean for Continuing Education, University of Texas HSC at Dallas; 5323 Harry Hines Boulevard, Dallas, Texas 75235; (214)688-2166.

RADECKI, Stephen E., Ph.D., Clinical Instructor of Medical Education, USC School of Medicine; 2025 Zonal Avenue, KAM 200, Los Angeles, California 90033; (213)224-7038.

REEVES, John, Ph.D., Loma Linda University Medical Center, 1911 South Commercenter East, Building 1, San Bernardino, California 92408; (714) 888-6434.

RICHARDSON, Penny, Ph.D., USC School of Education, University Park MC0031, WPH 701, Los Angeles, California 90089-0031; (213)714-2310.

ROSINSKI, Edwin F., Ed.D., University of California at San Francisco, 1356 Third Avenue, San Francisco, California 94143; (415)666-4102.

SCHWARTZ, Nancy E., Ph.D., University of British Columbia, School of Home Economics, Vancouver, B.C. V6T 1W5, Canada; (604)228-6874.

SHANNON, Michael, Ph.D., College of Pharmacy, University of Michigan; 1033 College of Pharmacy, Ann Arbor, Michigan 48109; (313)764-8053.

SHANNON, N. Fred, M.Ed., University of Washington, School of Medicine DORME SC 45, Seattle, Washington 98109; (206)543-2259.

SINOPOLI, Louis M., Ed.D., Evaluator, USC School of Medicine, Norris Medical Library, 2025 Zonal Avenue, Los Angeles, California 90033; (213)224-7038.

SMITH, Cheryl, M.S., New York City Technical College, 300 Jay Street/P514, Brooklyn, New York 11201; (212)643-5659.

STRAUSS, Marybeth, Ph.D., R.N., Ohio State University, School of Nursing, 1585 Neil Avenue, Columbus, Ohio 43210; (514)422-5371.

STUFFLEBEAM, Daniel L., Ph.D., Director of the Evaluation Center and Professor, Faculty of Education Leadership, Western Michigan University; Evaluation Center, Ellsworth Hall, Western Michigan University, Kalamazoo, Michigan 49008; (616)383-8166.

SULLIVAN, Toni J., Ed.D., R.N., USC Department of Nursing, Leavey Hall, 320 West 15th Street, Los Angeles, California 90089; (213)743-2362.

Figure 1–3 (continued)

TAYLOR, Joan P., Ed.D., Evaluator, USC School of Medicine, Norris Medical Library, 2025 Zonal Avenue, Los Angeles, California 90033; (213)225-7388.

UMAN, Gwen, R.N., M.N., Research Associate, Development and Demonstration Center, USC School of Medicine; 2025 Zonal Avenue, Los Angeles, California 90033; (213)224-7743.

WALSH, Patrick L., Ph.D., IRMC-Veterans Administration Medical Center (11-R), 500 Foothill Boulevard, Salt Lake City, Utah 84148; (805)582-1565, Ext. 1100.

WALTHALL, David III, M.D., Veterans Administration Medical Center, Continuing Education Center, 50 Irving Street N.W., Washington, D.C. 20422; (202)234-6080.

WEINSTEIN, Marvin, M.S., Associate Professor and Coordinator of Continuing Education, College of Pharmacy, University of Illinois; 833 South Wood Street, Room 138, Chicago, Illinois 60612; (312)996-7190.

WHITMAN, Neil, Ed.D., University of Utah School of Medicine, Department of Family and Community Medicine, 50 North Medical Drive, Salt Lake City, Utah 84132; (801)581-3614.

WOLF, Richard M., Ph.D., Professor of Psychology and Education at Teachers College, Columbia University, New York; 525 West 120th Street, New York, New York 10025; (212)678-3355.

WOLKOW, Muriel P., Ed.D., Director, Faculty Development Programs, Department of Medical Education, USC School of Medicine; 2025 Zonal Avenue, KAM 200, Los Angeles, California 90033; (213)224-7038.

YOUNG, Lynda, M.A., University of Minnesota School of Dentistry, 6-405 Health Science Unit A, 515 Delaware S.E., Minneapolis, Minnesota 55435; (612)373-7960.

Figure 1-3 (continued)

each of the first four subjects of the Conference. Chapter 2 is the presentation by Stufflebeam on the standards of educational valuation. Chapter 3 is the summary of participants' reactions to this first state-of-the-art presentation and is written by Burkett and Denson. Chapters 4 and 5 are Wolf's address on design issues followed by a summary of participant reactions by Martinoff.

Chapters 6 and 7 relate to Madaus's treatment of data collection and Nyquist's summary of practitioners' reactions. The next two chapters deal with data analysis, with the presentation by Cooley and the participant views by Hoffman. Finally, chapter 10 is the presentation by Abrahamson on the politics of evaluation; and chapter 11 is the conclusion, a summarization of the Conference by Joseph S. Green.

References

Abrahamson, S. (1968). "Evaluation in continuing medical education." *Journal of the American Medical Association*, 206(3), 625–628.

Bertram, D.A. and Brooks-Bertram, P.A. (1977). "The evaluation of continuing medical education: A literature review." *Health Education Monographs*, 5, 330–362.

Brown, C.R. and Uhl, H.S.M., Jr. (1970). "Mandatory continuing education: Sense or nonsense?" *Journal of the American Medical Association*, 213, 1660–1668.

Green, J.S. and Walsh, P.C. (1979). "Impact evaluation in continuing medical education — The missing link." In A. Knox (ed.), *Assessing the impact of continuing education*. New Directions for Continuing Education, No. 3. San Francisco: Jossey-Bass.

Green, J.S., Grosswalk, S.J., Suter, E. and Walthall, D.B. III (eds.). (1984). *Continuing education for the health professions: Developing, managing, and evaluating programs for maximum impact on patient care*. San Francisco: Jossey-Bass.

Lloyd, J. and Abrahamson, S. (1979). "Effectiveness of continuing medical education: A review of the evidence." *Evaluation and the Health Professions*, 2(3), 251–280.

Miller, G.E. (1967). "Continuing education for what." *Journal of Medical Education*, 42, 320–323.

Storey, P.B. (1978). "Mandatory continuing education." *New England Journal of Medicine*, 298, 1416–1418.

Walsh, P.L. (1981). "A Model for planning continuing education for impact." *Journal of Allied Health*, 10(2), 101–106.

Williamson, J. et al. (1967). "Continuing education and patient care research." *Journal of the American Medical Association*, 201(2), 118–122.

2 THE RELEVANCE OF THE JOINT COMMITTEE *STANDARDS FOR IMPROVING EVALUATIONS* IN CONTINUING EDUCATION IN THE HEALTH PROFESSIONS

Daniel L. Stufflebeam

Introduction

Continuing education has a vital role in assuring that health professionals provide services that are up-to-date and of high quality; and evaluations are needed both to examine critically continuing education and health services, and to provide direction for their improvement. Hence, evaluation has an important role in providing sound health care.

However, many things can and often do go wrong in evaluations: they are subject to bias, misinterpretation, and misapplication; and they may address the wrong questions and/or provide erroneous information. Indeed, there have been strong charges that evaluations of continuing education in the health professions have failed to render the services they are supposed to provide (Abrahamson, 1968; Brook et al., 1976; Bertram and Bertram, 1977; and Evered and Williams, 1980). Clearly, evaluation itself is subject to evaluation and to quality assurance efforts.

Since 1975, a joint committee appointed by 12 professional societies[1] has been conducting a systematic program by which to assure the quality of evaluation services in education. Their main product so far is a set of professional standards to guide and assess evaluations of educational programs, projects,

15

and materials (Joint Committee, 1981). Their ongoing assignment is to help promote the use of the Standards and to review and revise them. Their fundamental mission is to promote better education through sound evaluation.

The purpose of this chapter is to provide direction for using the *Joint Committee Standards* to improve evaluation services in continuing education in the health professions. In addition, it solicits feedback and assistance by which to improve the *Standards* and their applicability to continuing education in the health professions.

The chapter is divided into two parts: (1) an introduction to the *Standards*; (2) examination of the state of theory and practice of evaluation in continuing education in the health professions. Throughout, there are suggestions for using the *Standards* to upgrade evaluation practice.

Introduction to the Standards

In general, the Joint Committee devised 30 Standards that pertain to four attributes of an evaluation: Utility, Feasibility, Propriety, and Accuracy. The *Utility* Standards reflect the general consensus that emerged in the educational evaluation literature during the late 1960s concerning the need for program evaluations that are responsive to the needs of their clients, and not merely focused on the interests of the evaluators. The *Feasibility* Standards are consistent with the growing realization that evaluation procedures must be cost-effective and workable in real-world, politically charged settings; in a sense these standards are a countermeasure to the penchant for applying the procedures of laboratory research to real-world settings regardless of the fit. The *Propriety* Standards reflect ethical issues, constitutional concerns, and litigation concerning such matters as rights of human subjects, freedom of information, and conflict of interest. The *Accuracy* Standards build on those that have long been accepted for judging the technical merit of information, especially validity, reliability, and objectivity. Overall, then, the *Standards* promote evaluations that are useful, feasible, ethical, and technically sound — ones that will contribute significantly to the betterment of education.

Key Definitions

The *Standards* reflect certain definitions of key concepts. The object of an evaluation is what one is examining (or studying) in an evaluation: a program, a project, or instructional materials. Evaluation means the systematic investigation of the worth or merit of some object. Standards are principles commonly accepted for measuring the value or the quality of an evaluation. As I shall elaborate later, the definition of evaluation embodied in the *Standards* is considerably at variance with those which pervade the evaluation literature in continuing education in the health professions.

Development of the Standards

To ensure that the *Standards* would reflect the best current knowledge and practice, the Joint Committee sought contributions from many sources. They collected and reviewed a wide range of literature. They devised a list of possible topics for standards, lists of guidelines and pitfalls that they thought to be associated with each standard, and a format for writing each standard. They engaged a group of 30 experts to expand the topics and to write up alternative versions of each one. With the help of consultants, the Committee rated the alternative standards, devised their preferred set, and compiled the first draft of the *Standards*. They then had their first draft criticized by a nationwide panel of 50 experts who were nominated by the 12 sponsoring organizations. Based on those critiques, the Committee debated the identified issues and prepared a second draft. The project staff and Joint Committee reviewed this draft for correct and effective language, and developed a version which was subjected to national hearings and field tests. The results of these assessments led to the initial published version of the *Standards*. Presently, that version is being applied and reviewed, and the Joint Committee is collecting feedback for use in preparing the next edition.

The Developers of the Standards

An important feature of the *Standards*-setting process is the breadth of perspectives that have been represented in their development. The 12 sponsoring organizations include the perspectives of the consumers as well as those who conduct evaluation. The groups represented on the Joint Committee and among the approximately 200 other persons who contributed include, among others, those of statistician and administrator, psychologist and continuing education specialist, and theorist and school board member. There is perhaps no feature about the Joint Committee which is as important as its representative nature, since by definition a standard is a widely shared principle. However, just as the content of the *Standards* must be improved over time, so must there by continuing efforts to improve the representativeness of the participants in the standard-setting process. Clearly, there should be more representation from the health professions in the next revision cycle.

Format

The depth to which the Joint Committee developed each Standard is apparent in the format common to all of the Standards. This format starts with a *descriptor* — for instance, "Formal Obligation." The descriptor is followed by a *statement* of the Standard, i.e., "Obligations of the formal parties to an evaluation (what is to be done, how, by whom, when) should be agreed to in writing, so that these parties are obligated to adhere to all conditions of the agreement or formally to renegotiate it," and an *overview*, which includes a rationale for the Standard and definitions of its terms. Also included are lists of pertinent guidelines, pitfalls, and caveats. The guidelines are procedures that often would prove useful in meeting the Standard; the pitfalls are common mistakes to be avoided; and the caveats are warnings about being overzealous in applying the given Standards, lest such effort detract from meeting other Standards. The presentation of each Standard is concluded with an illustration of how it might be applied. The illustration includes a situation in which the standard is violated, and a discussion of corrective actions that would result in better adherence to the standard. Usually, the illustrations are based on real situations, and they encompass a wide range of different types of evaluations. One easy step to extending the applicability of the *Standards* to continuing education in the health professions would be to develop new illustrative cases drawn directly from experiences in evaluating continuing education in the health professions.

Content of the Standards

Utility Standards. In general, the Utility Standards are intended to guide evaluations so that they will be informative, timely, and influential. These Standards require evaluators to acquaint themselves with their audiences, ascertain the audiences' information needs, gear evaluations to respond to these needs, and report the relevant information clearly and when it is needed. The topics of the Standards included in this category are Audience Identification, Evaluator Credibility, Information Scope and Selection, Valuational Interpretation, Report Clarity, Report Dissemination, Report Timeliness, and Evaluation Impact. Overall, the Standards of Utility are concerned with whether an evaluation serves the practical information needs of a given audience.

Feasibility Standards. The Feasibility Standards recognize that an evaluation usually must be conducted in a "natural," as opposed to a "laboratory," setting and that it consumes valuable resources. The requirements of these Standards are that the evaluation plan be operable in the setting in which it is to be applied, and that no more materials and personnel-time than necessary be consumed. The three topics of the Feasibility Standards are Practical Procedures, Political Viability, and Cost Effectiveness. Overall, the Feasibility Standards call for evaluations to be realistic, prudent, diplomatic, and frugal.

Propriety Standards. The Propriety Standards reflect the fact that evaluations affect many people in different ways. These Standards are aimed at ensuring that the rights of persons affected by an evaluation will be protected. Especially, these Standards prohibit unlawful, unscrupulous, unethical, and inept actions by those who produce evaluation results. The topics covered by the Propriety Standards are Formal Obligation, Conflict of Interest, Full and Frank Disclosure, Public's Right to Know, Rights of Human Subjects, Human Interactions, Balanced Reporting, and Fiscal Responsibility. These Standards require that those conducting evaluations learn about and abide by laws concerning such matters as privacy, freedom of information, and protection of human subjects. The Standards charge those who conduct evaluations to respect the rights of others and to live up to the highest principles and ideals of their professional reference groups. Taken as a group, the Propriety Standards require that evaluations be conducted legally, ethically, and with due regard for the welfare of those involved in the evaluation as well as those affected by the results.

Accuracy Standards. Accuracy, the fourth group, includes those standards that determine whether an evaluation has produced sound information. These Standards require that the obtained information be technically adequate and that conclusions be linked logically to the data. The topics developed in this group are Object Identification, Context Analysis, Defensible Information Sources, Described Purposes and Procedures, Valid Measurement, Reliable Measurement, Systematic Data Control, Analysis of Quantitative Information, Analysis of Qualitative Information, Justified Conclusions, and Objective Reporting. The overall rating of an evaluation against the Accuracy Standards gives a good idea of the evaluation's overall truth value.

The 30 Standards are summarized in table 2–1.

Table 2-1. Summary Statements of the 30 Standards

A   Utility Standards
The Utility Standards are intended to ensure that an evaluation will serve
the practical information needs of given audiences.

A1   Audience Identification
Audiences involved in or affected by the evaluation should be identified so
that their needs can be addressed.

A2   Evaluator Credibility
The persons conducting the evaluation should be both trustworthy and
competent to perform the evaluation so that their findings achieve maximum credibility and acceptance.

A3   Information Scope and Selection
Information collected should be of such scope and selected in such ways as
to address pertinent questions about the object of the evaluation and be responsive to the needs and interests of specified audiences.

A4   Valuational Interpretation
The perspectives, procedures, and rationale used to interpret the findings
should be carefully described so that the bases for value judgments are clear.

A5   Report Clarity
The evaluation report should describe the object being evaluated and its
context, and the purposes, procedures, and findings of the evaluation so
that the audiences will readily understand what was done, why it was done,
what information was obtained, what conclusions were drawn, and what
recommendations were made.

A6   Report Dissemination
Evaluation findings should be disseminated to clients and other right-to-
know audiences so that they can assess and use the findings.

A7   Report Timeliness
Release of reports should be timely so that audiences can best use the reported information.

A8   Evaluation Impact
Evaluations should be planned and conducted in ways that encourage
followthrough by members of the audiences.

B   Feasibility Standards
The Feasibility Standards are intended to ensure that an evaluation will be
realistic, prudent, diplomatic, and frugal.

B1   Practical Procedures
The evaluation procedures should be practical so that disruption is kept to
a minimum and so that needed information can be obtained.

B2   Political Viability
The evaluation should be planned and conducted with anticipation of the
different positions of various interest groups so that their cooperation

Table 2-1 continued

---

may be obtained and so that possible attempts by any of these groups to curtail evaluation operations or to bias or misapply the results can be averted or counteracted.

B3   *Cost Effectiveness*
The evaluation should produce information of sufficient value to justify the resources expended.

C   *Propriety Standards*
The Propriety Standards are intended to ensure that an evaluation will be conducted legally, ethically, and with due regard for the welfare of those involved in the evaluation, as well as those affected by its results.

C1   *Formal Obligation*
Obligations of the formal parties to an evaluation (what is to be done, how, by whom, when) should be agreed to in writing so that these parties are obligated to adhere to all conditions of the agreement or formally renegotiate it.

C2   *Conflict of Interest*
Conflict of interest, frequently unavoidable, should be dealt with openly and honestly so that it does not compromise the evaluation processes and results.

C3   *Full and Frank Disclosure*
Oral and written evaluation reports should be open, direct, and honest in their disclosure of pertinent findings, including the limitations of the evaluation.

C4   *Public's Right to Know*
The formal parties to an evaluation should respect and assure the public's right to know, within the limits of other related principles and statutes, such as those dealing with public safety and the right to privacy.

C5   *Rights of Human Subjects*
Evaluations should be designed and conducted so that the rights and welfare of the human subjects are respected and protected.

C6   *Human Interactions*
Evaluators should respect human dignity and worth in their interactions with other persons associated with an evaluation.

C7   *Balanced Reporting*
The evaluation should be complete and fair in its presentation of strengths and weaknesses of the object under investigation so that strengths can be built upon and problem areas addressed.

C8   *Fiscal Responsibility*
The evaluator's allocation and expenditure of resources should reflect

Table 2-1 continued

sound accountability procedures and otherwise be prudent and ethically responsible.

D   *Accuracy Standards*
The Accuracy Standards are intended to ensure that an evaluation will reveal and convey technically adequate information about the features of the object being studied that determine its worth or merit.

D1   *Object Identification*
The object of the evaluation (program, project, material) should be sufficiently examined, so that the form(s) of the object being considered in the evaluation can be clearly identified.

D2   *Context Analysis*
The context in which the program, project, or material exists should be examined in enough detail so that its likely influences on the object can be identified.

D3   *Described Purposes and Procedures*
The purposes and procedures of the evaluation should be monitored and described in enough detail so that they can be identified and assessed.

D4   *Defensible Information Sources*
The sources of information should be described in enough detail so that the adequacy of the information can be assessed.

D6   *Valid Measurement*
The information-gathering instruments and procedures should be chosen or developed and then implemented in ways that will assure that the interpretation arrived at is valid for the given use.

D7   *Systematic Data Control*
The data collected, processed, and reported in an evaluation should be reviewed and corrected so that the results of the evaluation will not be flawed.

D8   *Analysis of Quantitative Information*
Quantitative information in an evaluation should be appropriately and systematically analyzed to ensure supportable interpretations.

D9   *Analysis of Qualitative Information*
Qualitative information in an evaluation should be appropriately and systematically analyzed to ensure supportable interpretations.

D10   *Justified Conclusions*
The conclusions reached in an evaluation should be explicitly justified so that the audiences can assess them.

D11   *Objective Reporting*
The evaluation procedures should provide safeguards to protect the evaluation findings and reports against distortion by the personal feelings and biases of any party to the evaluation.

Eclectic Orientation

The *Standards* do not exclusively endorse any one approach to evaluation. Instead, the Joint Committee has written *Standards* that encourage the sound use of a variety of evaluation methods. These include surveys, observations, document reviews, jury trials for projects, case studies, advocacy teams to generate and assess competing plans, adversary and advocacy teams to expose the strengths and weaknesses of projects, testing programs, simulation studies, time-series studies, checklists, goal-free evaluations, secondary data analysis, and quasi-experimental design. In essence, evaluators are advised to use whatever methods are best suited for gathering information which is relevant to the questions posed by clients and other audiences, yet sufficient for assessing a program's effectiveness, costs, responses to societal needs, feasibility, and worth. The methods should be feasible to use in the given setting.

Nature of the Evaluations To Be Guided by the Standards

The Joint Committee attempted to provide principles that apply to the full range of different types of studies that might legitimately be conducted in the name of evaluation. These include, for example, small-scale, informal studies that a continuing-education provider might employ to assist in planning and operating one or more workshops; as another example, they include large-scale, formal studies that might be conducted by a special evaluation team in order to assess and report publicly on the worth and merit of a program. Other types of evaluations to which the *Standards* apply include pilot studies, needs assessments, process evaluations, outcome studies, cost/effectiveness studies, and meta analyses. In general, the Joint Committee says the *Standards* are intended for use with studies that are internal and external, small and large, informal and formal, and for those that are formative (designed to improve an object while it is still being developed) and summative (designed to support conclusions about the worth or merit of an object and to provide recommendations about whether it should be retained or eliminated).

It would be a mistake to assume that the *Standards* are intended for application only to heavily funded and well-staffed evaluations. In fact, the Committee doubts whether any evaluation could simultaneously meet all of the Standards. The Committee encourages evaluators and their clients to consult the *Standards* to consider systematically how their investigations can make the best use of available resources in informing and guiding practice.

The *Standards* must not be viewed as an academic exercise of use only to the rich and powerful developers but as a code by which to help improve evaluation practice. This message is as applicable to those educators who must evaluate their own work as it is to those who can call on the services of evaluation specialists. For both groups, consideration of the *Standards* may sometimes indicate that a proposed evaluation is not worthy of further consideration, or it may help to justify and then to guide and assess the study.

Tradeoffs Among the Standards

The preceding discussion points up a particular difficulty in applying the *Standards*. Inevitably, efforts to meet certain Standards will detract from efforts to meet others, and tradeoff decisions will be required. For example, efforts to produce valid and reliable information may make it difficult to produce needed reports in time to have an impact on crucial decisions, or the attempt to keep an evaluation within cost limits may conflict with meeting such Standards as Information Scope and Selection and Report Dissemination. Such conflicts will vary across different types and sizes of studies, and within a given study the tradeoffs will probably be different depending on the stage of the study (e.g., deciding whether to evaluate, designing the evaluation, collecting the data, reporting the results, or assessing the results of the study). Evaluators need to recognize and deal as judiciously as they can with such conflicts.

Some general advice for dealing with these tradeoff problems can be offered. At a macro level, the Joint Committee decided to present the four groups of Standards in a particular order: Utility, Feasibility, Propriety, and Accuracy. The rationale for this sequence might be stated as "an evaluation not worth doing isn't worth doing well." In deciding whether to evaluate, it is therefore more important to begin with assurances that the findings, if obtained, would be useful, than to start with assurances only that the information would be technically sound. If there is no prospect for utility, then of course there is no need to work out an elegant design that would produce sound information. Given a determination that the findings from a projected study would be useful, then the evaluator and client might next consider whether it is feasible to move ahead. Are sufficient resources available to obtain and report the needed information in time for its use? Can the needed cooperation and political support be mustered? And, would the projected information gains, in the judgment of the client, be worth the required investment of time and resources? If such questions cannot be answered affirmatively, then the evaluation planning effort might best be discontinued with no further consideration of the other standards. Otherwise, the evaluator would next consider whether there is any reason that the evaluation could not be carried through within appropriate bounds of propriety. Once it is ascertained that a proposed evaluation could meet conditions of utility, feasibility, and propriety, then the evaluator and client would tend carefully to the accuracy standards. By following the sequence described above, it is believed that evaluation resources would be allocated to those studies that are worth doing and that the studies would then proceed on sound bases.

There are also problems with tradeoff among the individual Standards. The Committee decided against assigning a priority rating to each Standard because the tradeoff issues vary from study to study and within a given study at different stages. Instead, the Committee provided the Functional Table of Contents that is summarized in figure 2–1. This matrix summarizes the Committee's judgments about which Standards are most applicable to each of a range of common evaluations tasks. The Standards are identified down the side of the matrix. Across the top are ten tasks that are commonly involved in any evaluation. The checkmarks in the cells denote which Standards should be heeded most carefully in addressing a given evaluation task. All of the Standards are applicable in all evaluations. However, the Functional Table of Contents allows evaluators to identify quickly those Standards which are most relevant to certain tasks in given evaluations.

To assist evaluators and their clients to record their decisions about applying given Standards and their judgments about the extent to which each one was taken into account, the Committee provided a citation form (see figure 2–2). It is suggested that this form be completed, signed, and appended to evaluation plans and reports. Like an auditor's statement, the signed citation form should be of use to audiences in assessing the merits of given evaluations. Of course the completed citation form should often be backed up by more extensive documentation, especially with regard to the judgments given about the extent that each standard was taken into account. In the absence of such documentation, the completed citation form can be used as an agenda for discussions between evaluators and their audiences about the adequacy of evaluation plans or reports.

Validity of the Standards

In the short time since the *Standards* were published, a considerable amount of information that bears on the validity of the standards has been presented. In general, this evidence supports the position that the Joint Committee *Standards* are needed and have been carefully developed. However, the assessments also point out areas for improvement.

Standards (Descriptors)	1. Decide Whether To Do A Study	2. Clarify and Assess Purpose	3. Ensure Political Viability
A1 Audience Identification	X	X	X
A2 Evaluator Credibility	X		X
A3 Information Scope and Selection			
A4 Valuational Interpretation		X	X
A5 Report Clarity			
A6 Report Dissemination			X
A7 Report Timeliness			
A8 Evaluation Impact	X	X	X
B1 Practical Procedures			X
B2 Political Viability	X		X
B3 Cost Effectiveness	X	X	
C1 Formal Obligation	X		X
C2 Conflict of Interest	X	X	X
C3 Full & Frank Disclosure			
C4 Public's Right to Know			X
C5 Rights of Human Subjects			X
C6 Human Interactions			X
C7 Balanced Reporting			
C8 Fiscal Responsibility			X
D1 Object Identification	X	X	
D2 Context Analysis	X	X	
D3 Described Purposes & Procedures	X	X	X
D4 Defensible Information Sources			X
D5 Valid Measurement			
D6 Reliable Measurement			
D7 Systematic Data Control			
D8 Quantitative Analysis			
D9 Qualitative Analysis			
D10 Justified Conclusions			
D11 Objective Reporting			X

Figure 2-1. Citation Form

4. Contract the Study	5. Staff the Study	6. Manage the Study	7. Collect Data	8. Analyze Data	9. Report Findings	10. Apply Results
X		X			X	X
X	X	X	X			
X			X		X	
			X	X	X	X
					X	
X					X	X
X					X	
					X	X
			X	X		
X	X	X	X			X
		X				
X		X	X			X
X	X	X				X
X					X	
X					X	X
X		X	X			X
		X	X			
			X		X	X
X		X				
X			X	X	X	
			X	X	X	X
X		X	X		X	X
			X		X	
			X			
			X			
		X	X			
				X		
				X		
				X	X	X
	X				X	

Figure 2-1 (continued)

Citation Form*

The *Standards for Evaluations of Educational Programs, Projects, and Materials* guided the development of this (check one):

request for evaluation plan/design/proposal
evaluation plan/design/proposal
evaluation contract
other

To interpret the information provided on this form, the reader needs to refer to the full text of the standards as they appear in Joint Committee on Standards for Educational Evaluation, *Standards for Evaluations of Educational Programs, Projects, and Materials*. McGraw-Hill, 1980.

*The Publisher gives permission to photocopy this form.

The *Standards* were consulted and used as indicated in the table below (check as appropriate):

Descriptor	The Standard was deemed applicable and to the extent feasible was taken into account	The Standard was deemed applicable but was not taken into account	The Standard was not deemed applicable	Exception was taken to the Standard
A1 Audience Identification				
A2 Evaluator Credibility				
A3 Information Scope and Selection				
A4 Valuational Interpretation				

Figure 2-2. Citation Form

A5	Report Clarity			
A6	Report Dissemination			
A7	Report Timeliness			
A8	Evaluation Impact			
B1	Practical Procedures			
B2	Political Viability			
B3	Cost Effectiveness			
C1	Formal Obligation			
C2	Conflict of Interest			
C3	Full and Frank Disclosure			
C4	Public's Right to Know			
C5	Rights of Human Subjects			
C6	Human Interactions			
C7	Balanced Reporting			
C8	Fiscal Responsibility			
D1	Object Identification			
D2	Context Analysis			
D3	Described Purposes and Procedures			
D4	Defensible Information Sources			
D5	Valid Measurement			
D6	Reliable Measurement			
D7	Systematic Data Control			
D8	Analysis of Quantitative Information			

Figure 2-2 (continued)

Descriptor	The Standard was deemed applicable and to the extent feasible was taken into account	The Standard was deemed applicable but was not taken into account	The Standard was not deemed applicable	Exception was taken to the Standard
D9 Analysis of Qualitative Information				
D10 Justified Conclusions				
D11 Objective Reporting				

Name: _____   Date: _____

(typed)

Position or Title: _____

Agency: _____

Address: _____

Relation to Document: _____
(e.g., author of document, evaluation team leader, external auditor, internal auditor)

Figure 2-2 (continued)

Bunda (1982), Impara (1982), Merwin (1982), and Wardrop (1982) published papers in which they examined the congruence between the Joint Committee *Standards* and the principles of measurement that are embodied in the *Standards for Educational and Psychological Measurement* (1974); they independently concluded that there is a high degree of consistency between these two sets of standards with regard to measurement. Ridings (1980) closely studied standard setting in the accounting and auditing fields and developed a checklist by which to assess the Joint Committee effort regarding key checkpoints in the more mature standard-setting programs in accounting and auditing. In general, she concluded that the Joint Committee had adequately dealt with four key issues: rationale, the standard-setting structure, content, and uses. Wildemuth (1981) issued an annotated bibliography with about five sources identified for each *Standard*; these references help to confirm the theoretical validity of the *Standards,* and they provide a convenient guide to users of the *Standards* for pursuing in-depth study of the involved principles. Linn (1981) reported the results of about 25 field trials that were conducted during the development of the *Standards*; these confirmed that the *Standards* were useful in such applications as designing evaluations, assessing evaluation proposals, judging evaluation reports, and training evaluators. Additionally, they provided direction for revising the *Standards* prior to publication. Stake (1981) observed that the Joint Committee had made a strong case in favor of evaluation standards, but he urged a careful look at the case against standards. He offered an analysis in this vein and questioned whether the evaluation field has matured sufficiently to warrant the development and use of standards.

Several writers have examined the applicability of the *Standards* to specialized situations. Wargo (1981) examined the appropriateness of the *Standards* to federal program evaluations; he concluded that the Standards represent a sound consensus of good evaluation practice, but he called for more specificity regarding large-scale, government-sponsored studies and for more representation from this sector on the Committee. Marcia Linn, after her examination, concluded that the *Standards* contain sound advice for evaluators in out-of-school learning environments, but she observed that the *Standards* are not suitable for dealing with tradeoffs between standards or settling disputes between and among stakeholders. Nevo (1982) and Straton (1982), respectively, assessed the applicability of the *Standards* to evaluation work in Israel and Australia; they both concluded that while the *Standards* embody sound advice, they assume an American situation — regarding level of effort, citizen's rights, for example — that is different from their own national contexts. While the *Standards* explicitly are not intended for personnel evaluations, Lou Carey (1981) examined the extent to which they are congruent with state evaluation policies for evaluating teachers; she concluded that only one Standard (D11, Objective Reporting) was deemed inappropriate for judging teacher evaluations.

Four studies were conducted to examine the extent to which the *Joint Committee Standards* are congruent with the set of program evaluation standards that was recently issued by the Evaluation Research Society of America (1982). Cordray (1982), Braskamp and Mayberry (1982), Stufflebeam (1982), and McKillip (1983) found that the two sets of standards are largely overlapping.

Overall, the literature that has been developing on the *Joint Committee Standards* indicates considerable support for the *Standards*. They are seen to fill a need. They are judged to contain sound content. They have been shown to be applicable in a wide range of settings. They have been applied successfully. They are consistent with the principles in other sets of standards. And they are subject to an appropriate process of review and revision. At the same time, they have been shown to have limitations that need to be addressed in subsequent review and revision cycles.

The Guiding Rationale

The Joint Committee has been guided by a particular rationale in its efforts to develop and promote the use of the *Standards*. The benefits being sought include (1) a common language to facilitate communication and collaboration in evaluation, (2) general principles for dealing with a variety of evaluation problems, (3) a conceptual framework by which to study evaluation, (4) a set of working definitions to guide research and development on the evaluation process, (5) a public description of the state of the art in educational evaluation, (6) a basis for accountability by evaluators, and (7) an aid to developing public credibility for the educational evaluation field. These potential benefits are believed to be worth the investment of time and resources required to promulgate the *Standards*.

Nevertheless, there are certain risks in standard-setting efforts. These include promoting the establishment of a new field of professional practice that possibly is not needed, legitimating practices that may prove harmful, concentrating attention on matters of relatively little importance while diverting attention from major issues, inadvertently encouraging bad practices because they are not explicitly prohibited in the standards, and impeding innovation in evaluation. An account of the Joint Committee's assessment of these alleged risks as well as their plan to counteract risks deemed valid is contained in the *Standards* manuscript.

The preceding discussion of the *Standards* has been necessarily brief. The main intent has been to characterize the *Standards* sufficiently so that they can provide a framework for use in examining the state of evaluation practice in continuing education in the health professions.

Commentary on Evaluation Practice in Continuing Education in the Health Professions

From the perspective of the *Standards* and based on my experience and review of relevant material, I have developed a number of general impressions about the state of evaluation practice in continuing education in the health professions. The criteria that are accepted as appropriate for assessing evaluations in this domain are much narrower than those embodied in the Joint Committee's *Standards* and almost exclusively emphasize the value of technical adequacy. Corresponding to this narrow view of criteria for judging evaluations is the dominant tendency to define evaluation either as experimental research or as a determination of whether objectives have been achieved. Randomized experimental design clearly is seen as the method of choice. There has been substantial effort to define a wide range of variables and to employ practice-linked measures in assessing continuing-education programs. While differential continuing-education needs of individual health professionals are recognized in the continuing-education literature and in some instructional programs, they are rarely taken into account in evaluating the results of programs. It continually amazes me that many educators apparently see no contradiction in championing, on the one hand, programs that diagnose and address individual learning needs and, on the other hand, conducting evaluations that assess the worth of those programs based on the average scores on some group measure. Many evaluators in this field seem not to have distinguished between evaluations that are intended to guide program development and those that are oriented to assessing the overall value of a program, at least not in terms of the methods they use.

Also, I have seen little concern in this field for designing and conducting evaluations to foster improvement of programs; the concern seems to be almost exclusively one of proving the worth of continuing education. In this regard, evaluation in this field seems embroiled in an identity crisis: while the annual cost of continuing education in the health professions is counted in the millions of dollars, specialists in continuing education in the health professions are hard pressed to identify even one evaluation that has demonstrated the worth of an investment in continuing education. Not surprisingly, the main message in published reviews is that evaluations in continuing education in the health professions have rendered far too little valuable service.

The preceding impressions may seem harsh and careless. In the remainder of this part, I shall elaborate on them and cite my rationale. In so doing, I will refer to pertinent parts of the *Joint Committee Standards* and will attempt to offer suggestions as well as criticisms. I will illustrate my claims by referring to a particular evaluation drawn from the literature of continuing education in the health professions. In the spirit of the *Joint Committee Standard* labeled Balanced Reporting, I will underscore what I see as important strengths as well as weaknesses in existing views and practices of evaluation in continuing education. Finally, I acknowledge that my analysis is necessarily oversimplified, since there is obviously a diversity of viewpoints and practices in evaluation of continuing education in the health professions; but I believe I have correctly identified a dominant classicist position. In any case, I hope that my analysis at least will help to clarify the issues and to stimulate productive discussion.

An Illustrative Case

I chose an evaluation by Sibley and others (1982) as an illustrative case for examining strengths and weaknesses in evaluations of continuing education in the health professions. It is a well-known study and was carefully done. But it illustrates a number of the problems that plague evaluation.

In justifying the need for this study, the authors cited the annual multi-million-dollar cost of continuing medical education. They also charged that published evaluations of continuing education through the middle 1970s lacked rigor and did not satisfy the key criteria of validity and generalizability. In pursuing their own investigation they sought to test the assumption that continuing-education programs do more good than harm and that they help to improve the quality of health care. Their study was a randomized controlled trial in 16 general practices. They attempted to design and conduct the study to satisfy conditions of both internal validity and generalizability, but when tradeoffs had to be made they decided in favor of the former. For example, while they initially tried to select a representative sample from the identified study population for family physicians in Ontario, they ultimately chose 16 physicians from the ranks of the "eligible, consenting physicians." In their attempt to assure findings that would unequivocally assess cause-and-effect relationships, they randomly assigned eight physicians to a control group which received no special treatment and eight to an experimental group which received continuing education through the use of previously prepared self-instructional packets. At the outset, all 16 physicians were given a list of 18 educational packets and asked to rank their preferred four. The top two were assigned to each physician as "high-preference" conditions, and a systematic procedure was used to assign 2 of the 14 unranked packages as the "low-preference" conditions. Nurse-abstractors were trained and assigned to examine and code clinical records for each physician in relation to the two high-preference conditions, the two low-preference conditions, and two "hidden conditions." Pre-study measures of the quality of care were obtained from the control and study physicians. The previously selected self-instructional packets were provided to the treatment group. Subsequently, the posttreatment quality-of-care data were gathered and compared for the two groups.

Generally, Sibley and his colleagues reported that their findings were disappointing, and they concluded it is time to reconsider whether continuing education works. More specifically, they reported superior results for the treatment group in relation to low-preference conditions and no significant differences for the high-preference conditions and for all conditions combined. They observed that "continuing education programs that compel physicians to attend yet permit them to select their high-preference areas for instruction may represent the worst of both worlds" (Sibley et al., 1982).

While I make no claim that this case is typical or broadly representative of evaluation practice in the health professions, it is instructive. Also, it has generated considerable comment in the professional literature of medicine. Thus, I have used it in the remainder of this section to help identify key issues and to illustrate my points about strengths and weaknesses of evaluation practice.

Criteria for Judging Evaluations and Dealing with Conflicts

The study by Sibley and associates illustrates the importance of having in mind appropriate criteria for judging and guiding evaluation work. They invoked classical views of internal validity and external validity (Campbell and Stanley, 1963) both to assess the quality of prior evaluations and to guide the design of their own study. Unless inquirers invoke appropriate criteria for judging their study designs and reports, their studies are subject to a wide range of mistakes: addressing the wrong questions, producing misinformation, duping an uncritical audience, inviting criticism by hostile observers, and making the entire study vulnerable to attempts to discredit it, since the bases for defending it would not be clear. On the positive side, inquirers need appropriate criteria of sound investigation in order to review and rank alternative study designs, to monitor and guide the progress of a study, to assess and interpret results, and to provide direction for advancing the theory and practice of evaluation.

My criticism is not that evaluations of education have lacked a concern for appropriate criteria. It is that the scope of criteria employed often has been too narrow; I believe this narrowness has rendered much evaluation work in education useless or counterproductive.

As seen in the study by Sibley and colleagues, evaluators have often exclusively employed internal and external validity as the standards for judging their work. In general, internal validity calls for evaluations that produce unequivocal evidence about the effects of a program, and external validity calls for the use of settings and study samples that allow for defensible generalization to populations and contexts of interest. In short, internal and external validity assess the extent to which study designs and reports could or did produce sound and generalizable information.

Internal and external validity are consistent with the main thrust of the Joint Committee's Accuracy Standards, since these are also aimed at producing information which is technically defensible. But the Joint Committee has projected a much broader view of accuracy. They have assumed that treatments are much more complex, dynamic, individualized, and uncontrolled than those which are implied by conventional views on internal and external validity standards. Accordingly, the Joint Committee emphasized the importance of such additional principles as "logging and describing treatments in their various forms over time" (Described Object), examining and depicting the setting in which the treatment was observed (Context Analysis), evolving evaluation purposes and procedures so as to serve emergent as well as pre-established information requirements (Described Evaluation Purposes and Procedures), using multiple measures to ensure that outcomes are validly assessed (Valid Measurement), and systematically analyzing both qualitative and quantitative information. By taking into account the full range of the Accuracy Standards, an evaluator is required to consider programs as they evolve in real-world settings, to provide an in-depth multifaceted view of the programs, and to provide a variety of cross-checks so that the dependability of the information can be verified, without necessarily resorting to randomization and artificial laboratory controls.

Of course, exclusive concentration on internal and external validity takes no account at all of the Joint Committee's other three sets of Standards. As already argued, concerns for utility, feasibility, and propriety have a great bearing on whether a study should be conducted at all, and, if so, how it should be planned and carried through. The practice of "suboptimizing," i.e., concentrating exclusively on meeting internal and external validity criteria, is one way of dealing with conflicts and tradeoffs among competing standards, but it is a poor way. Inevitably, this approach to making tradeoffs must lead to decisions to proceed with studies without regard for their potential impact and in accordance with designs that are chosen regardless of the dynamic information needs of the relevant audiences, practical realities in the setting, and propriety considerations. Judging from some of the discourse in the literature of evaluation in continuing education in the health professions, there has been much such suboptimization and it has not infrequently led to field experiments that were later judged to have been unrealistic and to have yielded information of limited utility.

Evaluation: Research? Determining Achievement of Objectives? Assessment of Value?

Of course the issue of what criteria are appropriate for judging evaluations is tied to the fundamental issue of the meaning of evaluation. Whereas the Joint Committee drew on a common dictionary definition to characterize evaluation as "the systematic assessment of the worth or merit of some object," two somewhat more restricted definitions are commonly seen in writings on evaluation of continuing education in the health professions. One definition, implicit in much of the reported work (e.g., the study by Sibley and associates, 1982) equates evaluation with experimental research; the other characterizes evaluation as determining whether objectives have been achieved. I think these definitions are both flawed and dysfunctional for somewhat similar reasons.

Fundamentally, they skirt the central issue in evaluation which, of course, is *values*. Whereas an evaluation, by definition, must impute value or lack of same to some object, this is not merely a matter of ascertaining an effect of an intervention (as is appropriate in research investigations which are aimed at testing given hypotheses derived from a theory) or of determining whether it meets someone's objectives for it. An observed effect of treatment may be relatively meritorious or not depending on a wide range of factors, including the relevant guiding philosophy, the needs of the consumers, the possible existence of negative side effects, the performance of alternative treatments, the practical setting in which the treatment must be used, and the costs involved. Also, given objectives may or may not be an appropriate basis for judging outcomes; they may be unrealistic, too narrow, unreflective of assessed needs, or even immoral. In general, both of these definitions provide a focus for evaluation that is narrow and not directed to issuing comprehensive valuational interpretations.

Evaluation services in continuing education in the health professions could be greatly improved if evaluators and clients would appropriately conceptualize evaluation. Specialists in continuing education are professionals whose work is devoted to helping other professionals deliver high-quality services to the public. Assuring and demonstrating the value of such services are key roles of evaluation (Scriven, 1967). These roles must be implemented whether or not the evaluations produce any new knowledge through hypothesis-testing activity and whether or not the provider's goals are achieved. In many cases evaluations, rather than seeking new knowledge, should be oriented to determining whether continuing-education programs adequately translate existing theory and knowledge into practical application. Also, they should assess and rate outcomes irrespective of stated goals and, in fact, should judge whether the goals, as well as other structural aspects of a program, are realistic, appropriate, and otherwise worthy. Therefore, I propose that the field of continuing education in the health professions return to the fundamental meaning of evaluation. Evaluation is not research aimed at knowledge production, nor is it merely a determination of whether objectives have been achieved. Instead, it means ascertaining value, or assessing the worth and merit of a program or other object of interest.

Randomized Experimentation As Only One Way of Assessing an Educational Offering

Use of the definition proposed above would aid, I believe, in freeing continuing-education specialists in the health professions from what I see, all too often, as a slavish adherence to the use of randomized experiments as *the* method of evaluation. It would redirect the inquirer's attention to helping, through evaluation, first to attain valuable results and then to document and report relevant observations and judgments. Such an orientation requires the employment of a wide range of inquiry techniques, and, in general, a balanced approach to the use of both experimental and naturalistic methods.

An example drawn from my own realm of experience will help to illustrate the compulsive and frequently erroneous reliance on randomized experimentation. At a symposium, a well-known evaluator was describing his past efforts to develop a self-instructional manual on evaluation design. The manual was aimed at generalists in education, and the lesson to be learned was twofold: (1) evaluations should satisfy criteria of internal and external validity, and (2) the best means of doing this is through the use of randomized experiments. This evaluator described how he had taken his manual through a series of trials and revisions until trainees, after working through the manual, could consequently correctly identify internal and external validity as the appropriate criteria for judging evaluations, and, using these criteria, could select from several potential designs for a hypothetical study that one which most closely approximated a randomized experiment. In each development cycle, the evaluator had engaged about six educational administrators to work through the manual. He had then tested them against the objectives of the manual, had gathered their criticisms and recommendations, and subsequently had revised the manual. He was pleased to report that after about six developmental cycles, the manual had become so powerful that five of six participants could be expected to pass nine of the manual's ten test exercises.

However, this speaker wasn't prepared for one criticism. A member of the audience observed that the speaker's evaluation of the manual hadn't been directly oriented to satisfying conditions of internal and external validity and that the evaluation design employed most certainly hadn't been a true randomized experiment. Obviously embarrassed, the speaker acknowledged the shortcomings, cited some extenuating circumstances, and said that he would do better next time. His embarrassment was compounded when the critic rejoined that the speaker's evaluation performance had been somewhat better than his evaluation message: the administrators would have been better served, it was charged, by a functional and feasible approach to evaluation such as the one the speaker had actually used in his own developmental efforts. The critic qualified this observation, however, by noting that the evaluation had failed anyway, since it had helped to teach an erroneous message. These, indeed, were serious charges; if valid, the speaker had successfully used evaluation to brainwash his subjects.

This case helps to illustrate the interdependence of design, criteria for judging evaluations, and the definition of evaluation. Experimental design is not always a logical choice of method (the issue of design), especially if evaluation is needed to guide development (the issue of criteria for judging designs). But concentration on internal and external validity as the only criteria for use in selecting a study design might lead either to the choice of a design which would not yield the information needed or to inconsistency between one's espoused and actual practice of evaluation. And use of a restricted definition of evaluation, not oriented to assessing value, might lead one to judge a treatment as good because it effectively taught a developer's message, even though the message might be wrong.

The study of Sibley and associates (1982) provides another illustration of the hazards of overreliance on experimental design. By my assessment, and that of several other critics, the study was a weak evaluation of the instructional packages and of the overall approach they embodied. It employed static educational treatments; it substituted preferences for assessed needs; it expected dramatic effects based on small isolated treatments; and it attempted to generalize results based on the experiences of the small number of volunteer physicians. Seemingly, the investigators were so concerned with meeting the textbook requirements of an experiment that they neglected to develop and apply educationally sound treatments.

Barkin and colleagues (1982), by appealing to logic and educational theory, provided a more cogent assessment of the educational treatments than did Sibley and his colleagues. These critics questioned the conclusion by Sibley and associates that continuing medical education was ineffective and charged that they had failed to show changes in physicians' behavior in part because they had failed to apply and test educational techniques that have been shown to be effective in changing that behavior. Barkin and his colleagues contested the claim by Sibley and associates that the syllabi had been individualized. They charged that self-selection and uniform treatment characterized the design that was used. As seen in this criticism, an experimental design, once selected, can become a "Procrustean bed" which forces an educational program to fit the requirements of the design rather than ensuring that the evaluation will assist in developing an educational treatment that is likely to succeed in serving individual client needs.

Leonard Stein (1982) concurred. He compared the Sibley study to a 1980 report by White and others at the University of Iowa and charged that both groups erred in using preferences as their method of identifying needs. By contrast he cited eight studies published as a result of continuing medical education, and said that these programs differed in four educationally important ways from the treatments used by Sibley and colleagues. The continuing medical education was offered in a *clinical setting*; it focused on *problem-solving* with respect to current patients; its contents addressed the learners' *perceived needs* as well as objectively identified *gaps in performance*; and the participants were *fully involved* in designing the learning activities.

A more generalized critique of the experimental method has been provided by Bryk and Light (1981). They reminded us that uniformity constitutes the implicit assumption of all traditional univariate and multivariate analysis methods, and added that in contrast we have seen a concentration on individualized instruction. They concluded that traditional group-comparison designs that search for mean differences across groups are therefore futile. This is because "a highly individualized program can be effective without all of its subjects moving in a particular direction on all dimensions within a single evaluation time frame." A clear implication is that evaluators need to assess and count successes in terms that are relevant to each case. In a previous article (Stufflebeam, 1968) I projected a general design for gathering such individualized indicators of success, then aggregating and analyzing them so as to gauge the power of a program to meet individualized needs.

The foregoing discussion is intended not to refute the potential utility of the experimental method but to underscore its limitations and to point up instances of overuse and misuse. Under appropriate conditions, experimental design provides a powerful paradigm by which to gauge and demonstrate the power of a treatment. But experimentation is not a panacea; in many evaluative contexts it would be counterproductive and premature to compare educational treatments experimentally.

Developers must attend carefully to a variety of nonexperimental questions before it would make sense to impose experimental controls. They must assess the needs of individuals and groups to be served. They must carefully assess and evolve treatments that are responsive to these needs and that are otherwise educationally sound. They must develop a good deal of experience with the educational treatments, especially in clinical settings, and they should repeatedly try out, review, and revise the treatments until they, other observers, and the clients are convinced that the treatments are worthy of controlled testing. Then the developers and the evaluators could proceed with more confidence to demonstrate experimentally what they had already found in an applied setting to be true of their treatments. The emphasis in this scenario is first on the *development*, then on the *demonstration* of powerful treatments. It is consistent with the argument by Evered and Williams (1980) that "new techniques should be introduced only after rigorous evaluation in a pilot study has established a *prima facie* case for a more extensive experiment."

Varied approaches are needed to foster and demonstrate educational improvement. Fortunately, as stated earlier in this chapter, several techniques and models, in addition to the experimental-design approach, are available for use in evaluation work. *The Joint Committee Standards* — especially A3, Information Scope and Selection; A4, Valuational Interpretation; A8, Evaluation Impact; B1, Practical Procedures; D3, Described Purposes and Procedures; D4, Defensible Information Sources; D5, Valid Measurement; D8, Quantitative Analysis; and D9, Qualitative Analysis — provide a substantive guide for searching out, selecting, and applying a wide range of appropriate methods.

It is worth keeping in mind some warnings offered by Abrahamson and by Goldfinger. In commenting about the frustrations in past attempts to prove the worth of continuing education in the health professions, Abrahamson (1968) reviewed a broad range of potentially useful methods. But no matter how comprehensive the search for effects, he questioned whether it would ever be possible to attribute documented changes to specific continuing-education experiences. He said, "There are unfortunately so many intervening and contaminating variables that even the tightest experimental research design often leaves us frustrated in our attempt to establish cause and effect relationships." In a related view, Goldfinger (1982) argued that "if repetition and validation are essential components of a physician's effective learning, it may in the end be self-defeating to keep on examining single units of continuing education in order to find one that makes a substantial difference. Perhaps it would be more fruitful to recognize that contamination, a hindrance to studies of continuing medical education, is crucial to the process of learning and acting on one's knowledge." As Glass (1975) observed in his excellent essay on the "evaluation paradox," an overzealous effort to assess excellence may impede the pursuit of excellence.

Including Measures of a Wide Range of Potentially Relevant Variables

As Abrahamson (1968) observed, the success or failure of continuing education in the health professions is a function of many interacting variables. If evaluators are to contribute information that helps both to guide the development of effective continuing-education services and to assess what has been accomplished, then a wide range of variables must be taken into account. The literature of continuing education in the health professions is quite instructive about the range of variables that are potentially relevant for evaluation work in this domain. In general, the advice in this literature is consistent with that provided by the *Joint Committee Standards*, especially A3, Information Scope and Selection.

In their 1976 article, Brook and his colleagues made an important distinction between technical care and art of care. The former refers to the adequacy of the diagnostic and therapeutic processes; the latter, to milieu, manner, behavior, and communication. In a later publication, these authors (1977) presented a detailed taxonomy of potentially relevant variables for evaluating health services. In general, they argued that evaluations should provide information about structure, process, and outcome. They argued that many evaluations have erred by attending only to structure or process, and by assuming that strengths in these areas would automatically produce good results. They illustrated this point by saying, "The relationship between the medical care process itself and health status is not always direct. In many cases it may be so confounded by intervening variables such as patient compliance that adequate process may not result in good outcomes." While their taxonomy excludes the crucial area of needs, in general, they have made a substantial contribution by providing a rationale for the outcome method, linking it conceptually to assessment of structure and process, providing a taxonomy of variables, and applying it to eight disease conditions.

More directly related to continuing education is a review by Bertram and Bertram (1977). In reporting on the published evaluations of 66 continuing medical education programs, they observed that the variables measured included attendance, satisfaction, opinions, attitudes, knowledge, skill, physician behavior, and patient health status. Overall, then, evaluations of continuing education in the health professions evidence concern for a wide range of potentially relevant variables.

There is also evidence of some attention to practice-linked approaches to assessing continuing-education outcomes. In the study by Sibley and his colleagues (1982), physician performance was assessed by systematic analysis of clinical records. Mendenhall and his colleagues (1978) demonstrated the use of the Log Diary Technique. And Denson, Clintworth, and Manning (1983) collected and analyzed prescriptions as a basis for assessing a physician's individual needs for continuing education in the writing of prescriptions.

Such approaches to assessing applied performance are to be encouraged, but in most evaluations it is risky to rely too much on any one measurement approach. For example, the reliance in the Sibley study on analysis of patient records may have resulted more in an evaluation of the effects of the continuing-education program on physicians' keeping of records than on the patient care reflected in those records. Analysis of records may or may not be equivalent to assessing the performance that is supposedly reflected in the records. In general, triangulation — the assessment of a variable of interest by alternative methods — is to be encouraged so as to enhance the validity of the assessment.

Before leaving this discussion of measurement in evaluation studies, I wish to take issue with a particular view expressed by Brook and his colleagues (1976). They asserted, "In a sense, the concept of 'locally valid' outcome measures and process criteria is illogical or unjust and should not be pursued." They continued to maintain that "in the long run localism will be unacceptable because it almost guarantees development and acceptance of noncomparable (and potentially invalid) criteria and promotes uneven health behavior and outcomes." I have no quarrel with the practice of developing standardized instruments; in fact, that is a vital means of operationalizing and efficiently applying research-based measurement variables. But to focus exclusively on standardized measures and criteria is to ignore the fact that needs, philosophies, and approaches, as well as success criteria, may legitimately vary in a world of uncertainty. Also, these authors seem not to have considered that local solutions, while being potentially invalid, might also prove to be superior. If followed, the policy of invalidating localized measures and criteria would seem to lead to guaranteed mediocrity — standards that are appropriate in some settings, inappropriate in others, and a long-term drag on progress. Better advice, I believe, is embodied in the Joint Committee's Audience Identification and Information Scope and Selection Standards; they counsel a balanced approach which addresses variables that are theoretically important in assessing a certain type of program in addition to those that are of special interest to the particular audiences to be served by the evaluation.

Needs Assessment as a Basis for Focusing Services and Judging Outcomes

In general, educators have experienced little success in assigning value meaning to the findings of their evaluations. In experiments, the usual approach is to examine the statistical significance of observed differences between experimental and control groups; but the use of an arbitrary standard, such as a .05 alpha level, often begs the question of what levels of difference are excellent, good, bad, or indifferent. To their credit, Sibley and associates did attempt to define clinically important differences in quality of care, then choose an alpha level which, with about an 80 percent level of confidence, would identify differences at this level. Moreover, the typical analysis takes no account of the fact that a given level of effect may be more or less valuable to different participants depending on their particular aspirations and levels of performance.

Interpreting outcomes against pre-established objectives often is unsatisfying for much the same reasons. Objectives typically are based on predilections of the provider of education about what is important and on untested assumptions about the needs of the trainees. Usually the objectives are written for a group as a whole and are not differentiated to take account of individual differences. The predilections and assumptions of the educator may be defensible for the group as a whole, but almost certainly will prove inadequate in accounting for the aspirations and needs of individuals. Often the objectives are little more than rhetoric. Not infrequently, once a program is under way, pre-established objectives are pushed into the background and recalled only if a visiting authority wants to know what a program originally was intended to accomplish.

Two other approaches to valuational interpretation have proved even less useful. Few audiences are willing to defer to external evaluators for pronouncements about the quality of their work in the absence of clear-cut rationales and guidelines. Yet in my experience, they also are not satisfied if evaluators provide only descriptions without also including interpretations and recommendations. Leaving interpretation to the audience is considered by many clients to represent either benign neglect of duty or cowardice on the part of the evaluator; but giving authority for conclusions entirely to "the judge" at best is seen as risky.

Another approach, advocated by Robert Stake (1975), involves collecting, analyzing, and reporting the judgments of a wide range of interested persons. Using this approach, the evaluator reports findings to members of the audience and then collects their reactions, interpretations, and recommendations. These "judgments" are subsequently analyzed, summarized, and reported to take account of the represented value positions. The main advantages of this approach are that it is pluralistic (and sometimes democratic), and that it systematically involves the audience in interpreting the outcomes. Consequently, it promotes widespread communication about the findings and avoids the dominance of any particular bias. The weaknesses are that it is considered highly subjective, that it may be vulnerable to charges that the evaluator has pooled uninformed with informed judgments, and that it may confuse rather than provide clear direction.

The approach that I see as fundamentally most sound and potentially most useful is interpretation of results through the use of needs assessment. A physician's needs are assessed; an educational treatment designed to respond to these needs is delivered; and outcome data are gathered and interpreted against the assessed needs.

An example will help to clarify this approach. Over the past five years the University of Southern California (USC) Development and Demonstration Center has developed and offered a practice-linked approach to continuing education aimed at helping physicians improve their prescribing practice. In this "Office Education Project," each participating physician writes prescriptions for patients as usual, but on a special, slightly expanded form. After 200 have been written, copies are sent to USC, where a panel of experts reviews the prescriptions in order to identify what they see as errors or needs for improvement. The Committee then provides a clinical librarian with a report of identified needs for the given physician. The librarian prepares an individualized instruction packet for each need — including a statement of the need and corresponding objectives, examples of the offending prescriptions, and pertinent instructional material. After the physician has completed the individualized instruction packet, he or she collects 200 additional prescriptions and sends them to USC. The review panel, then, without being told the identity of the physician, reviews the prescriptions, again for the purpose of identifying needs or problems. If the needs for which the educational treatment was provided are still present, then — assuming that the estimate of needs was valid and that the review process was reliable — the educational treatment has to be judged a failure. But, if the same needs are no longer present and if the physician's patient population hasn't changed in any important ways, then a judgment of success for the continuing-education intervention is reasonable.

This approach to using needs to assign value meaning to findings has some important advantages. It judges success in terms that are relevant to each physician, and through an individualized approach to needs assessment it not only provides but validates "localized success criteria." At the same time, if the evaluator and client want to look at success in the aggregate or between experimental and control groups, the successes and failures can be quantified and combined to provide a judgment about the extent to which the set of individualized educational treatments resulted in meeting the previously assessed individual needs for improving prescribing practice. Another benefit of this approach is that the "posttest needs assessment" potentially provides direction for further individualized continuing education.

The Joint Committee Standard labeled Valuational Interpretation directs evaluators to document clearly and defend their approach to assigning value meaning to findings. That *Standard* refers to, but does not claim superiority for any of, the approaches mentioned above. I have advocated a needs-based approach; I also see merit in collecting and analyzing the judgments of different reference groups. And I see no reason why these two approaches shouldn't be used in concert. Clearly, the state of the art vis à vis valuational interpretation is primitive, and there is a need for research and development in this area. Perhaps the alternative approaches identified above are instructive about some developmental projects and comparative studies that might productively be pursued.

The Role of an Evaluation Study in Choosing Methodology

A number of writers have argued that evaluations are needed to serve different roles. Scriven (1967) distinguished between formative evaluation (that directed at guiding the development of a program or product) and summative evaluation (that designed to assess the worth and merit of something that has been developed and is ready for dissemination). Similarly,

Stufflebeam (1971) distinguished between evaluations intended to guide decision-making (the formative role) and those oriented to accountability (a summative role). Whatever labels one uses, different types of studies require different methodological approaches. The choice of method especially should be guided by the considerations found in all eight of the Joint Committee Utility Standards.

In my experience with evaluations of continuing education in the health professions, there is a predisposition to conduct a definitive experiment irrespective of the role to be served by the evaluation. Also there is too much of a tendency to view an evaluation as a single study aimed at uncovering and publishing a success story. Cronbach (1980) commented aptly on this problem: "Although sophisticated writers on evaluation are well aware that conclusions should be based on the cumulation of findings and not one single study, and aware that planning any one evaluation is more like planning a program of studies than a single focused test, the literature on design has not reflected this sophistication."

The study by Sibley and associates was deficient on these counts. The "treatment" they chose to test was not sufficiently flexible to respond to individual needs. Their sweeping conclusions about the ineffectiveness of continuing education were unwarranted, given their limited effort to develop responsive treatments and their failure to match treatments to needs. A more developmental approach could have yielded better results. It might have incorporated the following components: (1) identifying needs; (2) evolving responsive instructional offerings; (3) applying, observing, and revising these in clinical settings; (4) conducting some case studies; (5) involving the physicians in the search for effective instructional content and methods; (6) developing instrumentation and data-collection procedures to reflect the full range of effects against both collective and individual needs; (7) searching for cost-effective ways to deliver the service; and (8) demonstrating what has been learned through relevant experiments that take account of individualized needs and achievements. This long-term developmental approach might not have yielded publishable results any time soon. But in the long run I suspect it would have led to more satisfying services to physicians than did the experiment by Sibley and associates.

The Purpose of Evaluation: Not To Prove But To Improve

Fundamentally, I believe that continuing education in the health professions would be better served by evaluations that are oriented to *improving* continuing education and health care than by those designed to *prove* or *disprove* that continuing education has any beneficial effects. A number of arguments can be mounted in support of this position.

In any profession, the state of the art advances and its practitioners more or less continually assimilate and apply new developments. More pointedly, health professionals are and must be life-long learners. Continuing education is needed to facilitate the learning process and thereby to help assure that health care is up to date and of high quality. The most important role of evaluation in this context is to help ensure that continuing education services are focused on assessed needs, soundly conceived, and efficiently and effectively delivered. Efforts devoted to assessing whether continuing education should continue to exist are largely wasted, since realistically and philosophically this component of health care must endure. Evaluation dollars will be much better expended on efforts to help assure that continuing education excels in carrying out its vital role, than on summative assessments that do little more than cater to the field's identity crisis.

But care must also be taken to assure that evaluations contribute to and do not detract from the quality of both continuing education and of health care. Brook and others (1976), noting the arrival of quality assurance based on both federal and professional action, also pointed to its potential cost of 1 percent of each dollar spent on personal medical care, or about $2 billion annually. In considering this huge cost, they emphasized the need to raise questions about whether this expenditure will increase health levels by improving the quality of care provided or whether it will decrease health levels by transferring money that would provide new medical services to quality assurance efforts that lead to nonproductive activities.

This is a good example of what is at issue in the Joint Committee Standard B3, Cost Effectiveness. Evaluators should design and conduct studies that enhance, rather than detract from, services. If the projected influence of a study is not judged to be worth its cost, then it shouldn't be done. Otherwise it should be designed, financed, and conducted both to help improve continuing-education offerings and to help eliminate costly but unproductive continuing-education services. In this way evaluation services over the long term can be "cost free" (Scriven, 1974); i.e., they can help to save enough money (by eliminating unproductive services) to offset the costs of conducting the evaluations. Systematic application of the *Joint Committee Standards* in deciding when and how to pursue evaluations should aid greatly in assuring that allocations of funds for evaluations will result in the strengthening of beneficial continuing-education services and in the elimination of unproductive offerings.

One line of resistance to investing in evaluation of continuing education in the health professions is that the bottom-line evaluation of continuing-education services is seen in participation statistics. If participation remains high, then the services must be good enough and there is no need for systematic evaluation of the services. This is about as logical as concluding that medical services are as good as they should be so long as sick persons continue to seek the help of doctors. No, the hallmark of a professional is continual striving to improve services. Among other things, this means keeping up with the state of the art, striving to maintain the standards of the pertinent professional reference groups, and continually evaluating and upgrading one's contributions. An evaluation approach oriented to the improvement of services is highly appropriate within a professional context.

Scriven (1983) has emphasized that the commitment of a profession to evaluation should be pervasive. He wrote, "There is no such thing as professionalism without a commitment to evaluation of whatever it is that one supervises or produces — and to self-evaluation as well. Yet few professional schools have even the most superficial curriculum commitment to evaluation training of any kind."

Closing

In this chapter I have described the *Joint Committee Standards* and have presented my views about the state of evaluation theory and practice in continuing education in the health professions. I have also offered a number of suggestions.

Overall, I see a need to broaden the view of evaluation that is common in this field. The criteria used to plan and assess evaluations should be extended beyond those concerned with the technical merits of information. Evaluation should be defined to place primary emphasis on the assessment of value. Evaluators and their clients in this field need to escape the debilitating effects of overreliance on experimental design and should consider this as but one of a wide range of potentially applicable techniques. They should sustain their sound tradition of incorporating a broad range of variables and measurement approaches in their evaluations. They should devote more in-depth attention to assigning value meanings to findings, and in so doing should carefully distinguish between assessed needs and arbitrary standards such as objectives and levels of statistical significance. They should distinguish between formative and summative studies and should plan them accordingly. They would benefit much more from their evaluation investments if they would orient their studies to *improving,* as opposed to *proving the worth* of, continuing education.

The *Standards* provide an authoritative guide for effecting needed improvements. They offer a framework and pertinent content for offering training in evaluation. They likewise offer a comprehensive set of criteria for reviewing and assessing past evaluations; reviews based on the Utility, Feasibility, and Propriety Standards — as well as the Accuracy Standards — would no doubt yield insights well beyond those published by past reviewers who concentrated on internal and external validity. The *Standards* provide a checklist of considerations for decisions about whether to conduct a particular study and they offer in-depth advice for designing evaluations and judging reports.

Also, the Joint Committee is an organized, standing group that affords a forum for discussions and projects aimed at upgrading the theory and practice of evaluation in education. At present, no formal organization concerned with continuing education in the health professions is represented on the Joint Committee. Hence, there is no direct channel for input from and participation by this sector in the Standard-setting process. I encourage evaluators from the health professions to communicate with the Committee (c/o the Western Michigan University Evaluation Center) about how the *Standards* should be revised and used to promote sound evaluation in continuing education in the health professions. Also, the Committee would seriously entertain a recommendation to add a representative from the health professions.

Note

1. American Association of School Administrators, American Educational Research Association, American Federation of Teachers, American Personnel and Guidance Association, American Psychological Association, Association for Supervision and Curriculum Development, Council for American Private Education, Education Commission of the States, National Association of Elementary School Principals, National Council on Measurement in Education, National Education Association, and National School Boards Association.

References

Abrahamson, S. (1968). "Evaluation in continuing medical education." *Journal of the American Medical Association,* 206(3), 625–628.

American Psychological Association. (1974). *Standards for educational and psychological tests* (rev. ed.). Washington, D.C.: APA.

Barkin, Howard et al. (August, 1982). "Letter to the editor." *New England Journal of Medicine.*

Bertram, D.A. and Brooks-Bertram, P.A. (1977). "The evaluation of continuing medical education: A literature review." *Health Education Monographs,* 5, 330–362.

Braskamp, L.A. and Mayberry, P.W. (1982). *A comparison of two sets of standards.* Paper presented at the Joint Committee meeting of the Evaluation Network, Evaluation Research Society, Baltimore, Maryland.

Brook, R.H., Williams, K.N., and Avery, A.D. (1976). "Quality assurance today and tomorrow: Forecast for the future." *Annals of Internal Medicine,* 85(6), 809–817.

Brook, R.H., Davies-Avery, A.D., Greenfield, S., Harris, L.J., Lelah, T., Solomon, N.E., and Ware, J.E. (1977). "Assessing the quality of medical care using outcome measures: An overview of the method." *Supplement to Medical Care,* 15(9).

Bryk, A. and Light, R. (1981). "Designing evaluation for different program environments." In R.A. Beck (ed.), *Educational evaluation methodology: The state of the art.* Baltimore, Maryland: The Johns Hopkins University.

Bunda, M. (1982). *Concerns and techniques in feasibility.* Paper presented at the meeting of the National Council for Measurement in Education, New York.

Campbell, D.T. and Stanley, J.C. (1963). "Experimental and quasi-experimental designs for research on teaching." In N.L. Gage (ed.), *Handbook of research on teaching.* Chicago: Rand McNally.

Carey, L. (1979). "State-level teacher performance evaluation policies." *Inservice Centerfold.* Syracuse, New York: National Council on State and Inservice Education.

Cordray, D. (1982). "An assessment of the utility of the ERS standards." In P.H. Rossi (ed.), *Standards for evaluation practice.* New Directions for Program Evaluation, No. 15. San Francisco: Jossey-Bass.

Cronbach, L. and Associates. (1980). *Toward reform of program evaluation.* San Francisco: Jossey-Bass.

Denson, T., Clintworth, B., and Manning, P. (1983). *Final report of the office education project.* Los Angeles: University of Southern California Development and Demonstration Center.

ERS Standards Committee. (1982). "Evaluation research society standards for program evaluation." In P.H. Rossi (ed.), *Standards for evaluation practice.* New Directions for Program Evaluation, No. 15. San Francisco: Jossey-Bass.

Evered, D.C. and Williams, H.D. (1980). "Postgraduate education and the doctor." *British Medical Journal,* March, 626–628.

Glass, G. (1975). "A paradox about excellence of schools and the people in them." *Educational Researcher,* 4, 9–14.

Goldfinger, S.E. (1982). "Continuing medical education: The case for contamination." *New England Journal of Medicine,* 306(9), 540–541.

Impara, J.C. (1982). *Measurement and the utility standards.* Paper presented at the meeting of the National Council for Measurement in Education, New York.

Joint Committee on Standards for Educational Evaluations. (1981). *Standards for evaluation of educational programs, projects, and materials.* New York: McGraw-Hill.

Linn, R.L. (1981). "A preliminary look at the applicability of the educational evaluation standards." *Educational Evaluation and Policy Analysis,* 3, 87–91.

McKillip, J. and Garberg, R. *A further examination of the overlap between ERS and Joint Committee evaluation standards,* Unpublished paper, Southern Illinois University, Department of Psychology, Carbondale.

Mendenhall, R.C., Lloyd, J.S., Repicky, P.A., Monson, J.R., Girard, R.A., and Abrahamson, S. (1978). *Journal of the American Medical Association,* 240(11), 1160–1168.

Merwin, J.C. (1982). *Measurement and propriety standards.* Paper presented at the meeting of the National Council for Measurement in Education, New York.

Nevo, D. (1982). *Applying the evaluation standards in a different social context.* Paper presented at the 20th Congress of the International Association of Applied Psychology, Edinburgh, Scotland.

Ridings, J.M. (1980). *Standard setting in accounting and auditing: Considerations for educational evaluation.* Unpublished dissertation, Western Michigan University.

Scriven, M. (1974). "Evaluation perspectives and procedures." In W.J. Popham (ed.), *Evaluation in education: Current applications* (pp. 3–93). Berkeley: McCutchan.

Scriven, M. (1983). Evaluation ideologies." In G.F. Madaus, M. Scriven, and D.L. Stufflebeam (eds.), *Evaluation models.* Hingham, Massachusetts: Kluwer-Nijhoff Publishing.

Sibley, J.C., Sackett, D.L., Neufeld, V., Gerrard, B., Rudnick, K.V., and Fraser, W.A. (1982). "Randomized trial of continuing medical education." *New England Journal of Medicine,* 306, 511–515.

Stake, R. (1975). *Program evaluation, particularly responsive evaluation.* (Occasional Paper Series, No. 5). Kalamazoo: Western Michigan University Evaluation Center.

Stake, R. (1981). "Setting standards for educational evaluators." *Evaluation News,* 2(2), 148–152.

Stein, L. (August 19, 1982). "Letter to the editor." *New England Journal of Medicine.*

Straton, R.B. (1982). *Appropriateness and potential impact of programme evaluation standards in Australia.* Paper presented at the 20th International Congress of Applied Psychology, Edinburgh, Scotland.

Stufflebeam, D.L. (1968). "The use of experimental design in educational evaluation. *Journal of Educational Measurement,* 8(4), 267–274.

Stufflebeam, D.L. et al. (1971). *Educational evaluation and decision making.* Itasca, Illinois: F.E. Peacock.

Stufflebeam, D.L. (1982). *An examination of the overlap between ERS and Joint Committee standards.* Paper presented at the Annual Meeting of the Evaluation Network, Baltimore, Maryland.

Wardrop, J.C. (1982). *Measurement and accuracy standards.* Paper presented at the meeting of the National Council for Measurement in Education, New York.

Wargo, M.J. (1981). "The standards: A federal level perspective." *Evaluation News,* 2(2), 157–162.

Wildemuth, B.M. (1981). A bibliography to accompany the Joint Committee's standards on educational evaluation. (ERIC/TM, Report 81). Princeton, New Jersey: Educational Testing Service.

3 ANOTHER VIEW OF THE STANDARDS

Deborah Burkett and Teri Denson

Introduction

This chapter is divided into three sections. The first section is based upon reactions from Conference participants to Stufflebeam's presentation on "The Relevance of the Standards for Improving Evaluations in Continuing Education in the Health Professions." In general, participant comments were not addressed to specific points raised by Stufflebeam; rather, they served to focus attention on the perceived needs of evaluators in the health-professions education field and helped to identify areas for which the *Standards* met or fell short of the expectations of those evaluators in attendance.

The second section of this chapter represents an attempt by the Conference organizers to address a crucial substantive issue raised by participants: the distinction between small-scale and large-scale evaluation projects. Specifically, a survey was undertaken among Conference "recappers" (who were also evaluators in the health-professions-education field) to identify those *Standards* which would be most applicable to both small-scale and large-scale evaluations.

The last section provides a one-page recap of key points made by Stufflebeam.

Participant Comments

In response to Stufflebeam's presentation, there was a general recognition on the part of the Conference participants that the *Standards* represent a useful framework for designing evaluations and offer substantial potential for application to the evaluation of continuing education (CE) programs for the health professions. Participants agreed with the point that evaluators cannot apply all of the *Standards* equally well in all evaluation projects but must select those *Standards* that are most applicable for a given problem. At issue, for most participants, was how an evaluator goes about the task of identifying those *Standards* which will allow them to maximize the evaluation process and minimize factors which may undermine the evaluation. A number of criticisms and recommendations regarding the *Standards* were made by participants. These issues have been organized and summarized under one of the following themes: (1) State of the art versus state of affairs; (2) scope of the *Standards*; and (3) applicability of the *Standards* to health professions education.

State of the Art Versus State of Affairs

One difference between the state of the art and the state of affairs that emerged in group discussions is that the *Standards*, which were designed to be used by evaluators, contain crucial elements that tend to lie outside the evaluator's professional area of control, particularly those in the area of corporate or institutional policy. Although some of the *Standards* may appear reasonable from the evaluator's point of view, implementation may not be entirely feasible. Thus, any attempts to apply the state of the art in educational evaluation within a rigidly stratified institutional setting may be rendered ineffective by higher-level decisions.

Since many of the Conference participants were staff evaluators for multiple small-scale projects or courses, issues such as the identification of the purposes of the evaluation or even the determination of questions to be asked often did not fall within their jurisdiction. Typically, instruments used for data collection in course evaluations, for example, already exist within an organization. In addition, the evaluator's superiors expect these to be used routinely with little or no opportunities for modifications.

Another point of concern, pointed out by Conference participants, was that the *Standards* focused on the evaluator as someone who is external to the project, when very often the person administering the program is also expected to evaluate it.

Scope of the Standards

Many Conference participants indicated that Stufflebeam's presentation, as well as the open discussion that followed, focused on heavily funded, long-term projects and virtually disregarded small-scale projects. It became apparent that those in attendance included two distinct groups of evaluators: those who were experienced in evaluating large-scale, long-term projects and those who were expected to evaluate numerous, small-scale, short-term projects. It was suggested by some of the participants that a separate set of *Standards* may be needed — one each for large-scale and small-scale evaluations.

Other participant suggestions included (1) that the *Standards* be put in a "functional" order rather than in alphabetical order, so that they would follow the same sequence in which a research project normally unfolds; and (2) that the *Standards* incorporate bibliographic references that would provide more examples of direct applications of the Standards.

There was also considerable discussion among participants regarding the language used in some of the Standards as being too broad, and in need of clarification in some areas. As an example, with reference to the first Standard, A1, Audience Identification,[1] the general consensus of the small groups was that the definition of "audience" was too broad — "so broad, that it basically included everybody in the world who might ever be involved in, or have any impact on the evaluation."

Participants indicated that more guidelines were called for to describe how to narrow the scope of the audience, and particularly to clarify the basis upon which an evaluator begins to prioritize his or her audiences. In addition, several groups called for guidelines for clarifying the time at which a given audience should become involved in the evaluation process. Still other participants felt that Standard A1 did not clarify the distinction an evaluator must make between subjects from whom the data are collected and those who use the data once they have been generated.

Another Standard[2] was also considered too broad to be useful for CE evaluations in the health-professions field. Participants indicated that more guidelines were needed to illuminate the process of *how* to determine what information is essential to a sound evaluation and what strategies are most useful in eliminating minor information.

Applicability of the Standards to Health Professions Education

Although, in general, Conference participants recognized the potential value of needs assessment in applying the *Standards* to the evaluation of continuing-education programs in the health field, there were some reservations expressed concerning the appropriate focus of that assessment. In the health field, as in other professions, the ultimate outcome of an educational intervention affects not only the client of the evaluation but also the patient and his or her health, happiness, and satisfaction with the care received. But the needs and desires of the patient may differ from what the health professional feels is in the patient's best interest. Therefore, a comprehensive needs assessment must go beyond the gathering of information on client needs and extend into the ultimate goal of the maintenance or improvement of the patient's health. Thus, to become fully applicable to the health professions, the *Standards* must incorporate a type of needs assessment that goes beyond that used for the typical client of an educational intervention and extend into projected outcomes for that successful intervention.

In addition, it was recommended that illustrative cases drawn directly from health-related situations would be more useful to the health professions educational evaluators than public school applications to which the *Standards* text is addressed.

Appropriateness of the *Standards* for Large-Scale and Small-Scale Evaluations

Definitions

Growing out of the participants' expressed interest in using the Standards to evaluate continuing education in the health-professions education field, it was considered important to adapt the *Standards* to the health professions. First of all, it was necessary to make a distinction between large-scale and small-scale evaluation projects. The following definitions were developed.

> *Large-Scale:* Formal studies that are conducted by a special evaluation team to assess and report publicly on the worth and merit of a program. Usually externally funded, the major purpose of such an evaluation is to develop, demonstrate, or test the effectiveness of an educational intervention.
> *Small-Scale:* Informal studies that a CE provider employs to assist in planning and operating one or more programs. These are locally initiated and provide only limited learning experiences for participants.

Method

In an effort to identify the most appropriate Standards for both large-scale and small-scale evaluations, and taking into consideration time constraints structured by the Conference itself, six experienced health-professions education evaluators, who served as recappers for the small-group discussions, were chosen as individuals who had extensive field experience in evaluating both large-scale and small-scale continuing-education programs in the health-professions education field. Each respondent was provided with a packet that consisted of three parts: (1) a cover letter describing the details of the survey; (2) definitions of small-scale and large-scale evaluations; and (3) a survey instrument. The survey instrument included two sections. The first section listed 30 Standards, each of which was to be considered in terms of its appropriateness for small-scale evaluations only. The second section also listed the 30 Standards, each to be considered in terms of its appropriateness for large-scale evaluations. Respondents were directed to indicate the extent to which each of the Standards was important at each of four general stages in the evaluation process: (1) design, (2) data collection, (3) analysis, and (4) reporting. A six-point rating scale was provided for each item, with the number 1 indicating a "not important" Standard when applied to small-scale (or large-scale) evaluations, and number 6 identifying a "vitally important" Standard.

Results

Completed surveys were reviewed and responses tabulated. Only those Standards that were identified by respondents as applicable and "important" or "vitally important" to both large-scale and small-scale evaluations are shown in table 3–1.

Table 3–1. Standards Identified as Important for Both Large-Scale and Small-Scale Evaluation Projects

	Standard	*Application Area*
A1	Audience Identification	Design
A2	Object Identification	Design
B1	Practical Procedures	Data collection
C5	Rights of Human Subjects	Data collection
D9	Analysis of Qualitative Information	Analysis
D8	Analysis of Quantitative Information	Analysis
D10	Justified Conclusion	Analysis
D7	Systematic Data Control	Analysis
A5	Report Clarity	Reporting
C3	Full and Frank Disclosure	Reporting

Recap of Key Points from Stufflebeam's Presentation

The *Standards* are offered as suggestions and guidelines, not axioms. Secondly, the *Standards* are grouped in a particular order to facilitate decision-making for the evaluator[3]:

1. Utility Standards — " . . . if there is no prospect for utility (that the findings are useful) . . . there is no need to work out an elegant design."
2. Feasibility Standards — " . . . if findings from a projected study would be useful then . . . are sufficient resources available (to get the job done)? . . . can needed cooperation and political support be mustered . . . ? And, would the . . . gains . . . be worth the time and resources (to the client)?"
3. Propriety Standards — " . . . can the evaluation . . . be carried through within appropriate bounds of propriety?"
4. Accuracy Standards — does the design and the instrumentation incorporate appropriate tests of reliability, validity, and other measures of "objectivity" to assure the technical merit of the study?

Notes

1. *Standard A1:* Audiences involved in or affected by the evaluation should be identified so that their needs can be addressed.
2. *Standard A3:* Information collected should be of such scope and selected in such ways as to address pertinent questions about the object of the evaluation and be responsive to the needs and interests of specified audiences.
3. A Functional Table of Contents for the *Standards* has been provided by the Joint Committee to "help evaluators quickly identify those Standards which are most relevant to certain tasks in given evaluations."

4 DESIGN PROBLEMS IN EVALUATION

Richard M. Wolf

A great man died in the summer of 1982. His name was William McCall. Throughout his life, McCall made a number of important contributions to the field of education. He invented the T-Score, developed tests and teaching materials, and conducted a number of important educational studies. In 1923, McCall published *How to Experiment in Education*, the first systematic application of experimental procedures to the field of education. Campbell and Stanley (1963), in their now-classic chapter on "Experimental and Quasi-Experimental Designs in Research and Teaching," acknowledge their debt to McCall by stating, at the outset, that their chapter was merely an updating of ideas propounded by McCall. I can assure you that they were not suffering from excessive modesty.

McCall's book made two major points. First, judgments about the efficacy of educational treatments should be based on empirical studies rather than debate; second, such studies should be carried out in the field rather than in laboratory settings. McCall's book proceeded to set forth how this could be done. Both points were important ones for the time. There was, and in some quarters still is, a strong impulse to decide issues of the effectiveness of educational treatment through argumentation rather than on the basis of evidence. McCall argued forcefully for the latter. McCall's second point was more subtle. By the 1900s, psychology had established itself as a science, and there was a developing tradition that laboratory studies furnished the major way of producing knowledge. The legacy of Wilhelm Wundt and his coworkers in Leipzig had set a strong experimental tradition for psychology. Laboratory conditions, it was argued, provided the best and, really, the only way of controlling all relevant variables so that causal inferences could be made. McCall questioned and rejected this view. His contention was that the generalization of laboratory results to real settings was not automatic and, in the case of education, downright dubious. The path to knowledge, McCall argued, lay in doing the best possible job of studying the effects of educational treatments in real settings and trying to control conditions as best one could. It evidenced a major concern for external validity. It is interesting to note how, in 60 years, we have come full circle to what McCall advocated.

Before tracing the development of ideas from the time McCall's book was published to the present, it is necessary to review a few basic ideas about study design. In educational studies one is concerned with the causal effect that a treatment (T) such as continuing medical education has on performance (P). This is represented by the diagram below in which the arrow denotes a causal influence.

$$T \longrightarrow P$$

A number of people have problems with the notion of causation and tend to become enmeshed in the philosophy of science. Some even lose their way in the works of Locke, Hume, Kant, Mill, Russell, and Popper, never to be heard from again. An obsession with causation will be avoided here by simply noting that causal assertions are meaningful at a molar level even though we may not know the precise mechanisms by which an effect results from a cause. For example, a young child entering a dark room flips the light switch to illuminate the room even though he or she may know next to nothing about electron flow, switching mechanisms, and electrical resistance in a vacuum.

In the diagram above, one may postulate that the treatment is some program of continuing medical education and the performance is increased physician knowledge and/or competence (skills, diagnostic ability, etc.). As one reads the literature on continuing medical education, however, one is struck by the fact that the implicit model involved something more than the simple $T \longrightarrow P$. My sense of that model is that it is as follows:

Continuing Medical Education		Increased Physician Competence		Improved Physician Performance		Improved Patient Health Status
	$\longrightarrow$		$\longrightarrow$		$\longrightarrow$	

This is a complex causal chain which I believe serves as the basic rationale for continuing medical education and for programs of continuing education for other health professionals. Whether it can be fully tested is open to question.

In an experimental study, one wishes to be able to say that the introduction of an educational treatment is always followed by a particular resulting performance level. Of course, this never happens. Molar causal effects, because they are contingent on many other conditions and causal laws, are fallible and hence probabilistic. Again, this need not cripple us in our endeavors. We are content, if not ecstatic, to be able to say that if I give program X to a group of physicians it will most likely be followed by a particular (increased) level of knowledge and skill. Note the use of the phrase "most likely" instead of the word "inevitably." Continuing education programs in the health professions, like all educational programs, must be viewed *probabilistically* rather than *deterministically* — just as the actual practice of medicine is probabilistic.

Internal Validity

In order to establish a causal influence, it is equally important to be able to say that a particular performance (outcome) was *not* due to some other event or set of events as to say it was because of the educational treatment under study. For example, if a program of continuing medical education on pityriasis rubra were instituted in a particular setting and many of the physicians who attended the program also received personal visits from a drug company representative who talked with them at length about pityriasis rubra and gave them a considerable amount of printed material along with samples of a new drug to control it, then it is obviously questionable whether increased physician knowledge about pityriasis rubra was due solely to the effects of the continuing-education program. In fact, there is at least one highly plausible alternative hypothesis as to what brought about the increased level of physician knowledge.

Internal validity refers to the fact that the effects of a treatment are due to the power of the treatment and not to *something else*. Any equivocation on this matter means that there are one or more alternative explanations for a set of obtained effects. In the nomenclature of research design, these are called threats to internal validity. Cook and Campbell (1979) have set forth a rather comprehensive list of such threats. Some that are particularly relevant for studies in continuing medical education include the following:

1. History

"History" is a threat when an observed effect might be due to an event which takes place between the pretest and the posttest, when this event is not the treatment of research interest. In much laboratory research the threat is controlled by insulating respondents from outside influences (e.g., in a quiet laboratory) or by *choosing dependent variables* that could not plausibly have been affected by outside forces (e.g., the learning of nonsense syllables). Unfortunately, these techniques are rarely available to the field researcher.

2. Testing

This is a threat when an effect might be due to the number of times particular responses are measured. In particular, familiarity with a test can sometimes enhance performance because items and error responses are more likely to be remembered at later testing sessions.

3. Instrumentation

This is a threat when an effect might be due to a change in the measuring instrument between pretest and posttest and not to the treatment's differential impact at each time interval. Thus, instrumentation is involved when human observers become more experienced between a pretest and posttest or when a test shifts in metric at different points. The latter can happen, for instance, if intervals are narrower at the ends of a scale than at the midpoint, resulting in so-called ceiling or basement effects. (Basement effects are also called "floor" effects.)

4. Statistical Regression

This is a threat when an effect might be due to respondents being classified into experimental groups at, say, the pretest on the basis of pretest scores or correlates of pretest scores. When this happens and measures are unreliable, high pretest scorers will score relatively lower at the posttest and low pretest scorers will score higher. It would be wrong to attribute such differential "change" to a treatment because it might be due to statistical regression.

Viewed more generally, statistical regression (1) operates to increase obtained pretest–posttest gain scores among low pretest scores, since this group's pretest scores are more likely to have been depressed by error; (2) operates to decrease obtained change scores among persons with high pretest scores since their pretest scores are likely to have been inflated by error; and (3) does not affect obtained change scores among scorers at the center of the pretest distribution since the group is likely to contain as many units whose pretest scores are inflated by error as units whose pretest scores are deflated by it. Regression is always to the population mean of a group. Its magnitude depends both on the test–retest reliability of a measure and on the difference between the mean of a deliberately selected subgroup and the mean of the population from which the subgroup was chosen. The higher the reliability and the smaller the difference, the less will be the regression.

5. Selection

This is a threat when an effect may be due to the difference between the kinds of people in the experimental group as opposed to a comparison group. Selection is therefore pervasive in quasi-experimental research, which is defined in terms of different groups receiving different treatments as opposed to probabilistically equivalent groups receiving treatments as in the randomized experiment.

6. Mortality

This is a threat when an effect may be due to the different kinds of persons who dropped out of a particular treatment group during the course of an experiment. This results in a selection artifact, since the groups are then composed of different kinds of persons at the posttest.

7. Interactions with Selection

Many of the foregoing threats to internal validity can interact with selection to produce forces that might spuriously appear as treatment effects. Among these are selection-history and selection-instrumentation. Selection-history (or local history) results from the various treatment groups coming from different settings so that each group could experience a unique local history that might affect outcome variables. (The interaction can also occur with randomized experiments if a treatment is only implemented at one or two sessions — usually with large groups of respondents. In such cases, the treatment will be associated with any unique events that happened during the few sessions which provided all the data about a particular treatment's effects.) Selection-instrumentation occurs when different groups score at different mean positions on a test whose intervals are not equal. The best-known examples of this occur when there are differential "ceiling" and "floor" effects, the former being when an instrument cannot register any more true gain in one of the groups, and the latter when more scores from one group than another are clustered at the lower end of the scale.

8. Diffusion or Imitation of Treatments

When treatments involve informational programs and when the various experimental (and control) groups can communicate with each other, respondents in one treatment group may learn the information intended for others. The experiment may, therefore, become invalid because there are no planned differences between experimental and control groups. This problem may be particularly acute in quasi-experiments where the desired similarity of experimental units may be accompanied by a physical closeness that permits the groups to communicate. For example, if a new program of continuing medical education were tried out in a particular county and no attempts were made to have program participants withhold program materials and notes from nonparticipants, any true effects of the program could be obscured through the sharing that went on.

9. Resentful Demoralization of Respondents Receiving Less Desirable Treatments

When an experiment is obtrusive, the reaction of a no-treatment control group or groups receiving less desirable treatments can be associated with resentment and demoralization. This is because persons in the less desirable treatment groups are often relatively deprived when compared to others. In an industrial setting the persons experiencing the less desirable treatments might retaliate by lowering productivity and company profits, while in an educational setting, teachers or students could "lose heart" or become angry and "act up." Any of these forces could lead to a posttest difference between treatment and no-treatment groups, and it would be quite wrong to attribute the difference to the planned treatment. Cause would not be from the planned cause, T, given to a treatment group. Rather, it would be from the inadvertent resentful demoralization experienced by the no-treatment controls (adapted from Cook and Campbell, 1979, pp. 51–55).

The purpose of study design is to control the scheduling of individuals, treatments, and observations or measurements in such a way that threats to internal validity are effectively removed. The two major ways of achieving such control are (1) randomization, and (2) the use of standard procedures and instruments. When participants are randomly assigned to groups and groups are randomly assigned to treatment condition, each group is similarly constituted on the average (no selection problems). Each group experiences the same testing conditions and research instruments (no testing or instrument problems). No deliberate selection is made of high and low scorers on any tests except under conditions where respondents are first matched according to, say, pretest scores and then randomly assigned treatment conditions (no statistical regression problem). Each group experiences the same global pattern of history (no history problem). And if there are treatment-related differences in those who drop out of the study, this is interpretable as a consequence of the treatment. Thus, randomization and the use of standard procedures and instruments take care of many threats to internal validity. Schematically, this situation can be represented as

$$\boxed{R} \quad \frac{P \quad T \quad P}{P \qquad P}$$

where R denotes randomization, P denotes performance measures, and T denotes the presence of a treatment. The line in the schema distinguishes between the two groups studied: the treatment and the no-treatment control groups.

Campbell and Stanley (1963) call this design a classic true experiment. The use of randomization procedures combats most of the threats to internal validity. In their chapter, Campbell and Stanley strongly advocated the use of this and similar designs in which procedures of randomization were used. In contrast, quasi-experimental designs lack randomization and, consequently, do not furnish the assurance of comparability between groups that randomization does. Unfortunately, many readers of Campbell and Stanley's chapter erroneously concluded that true experiments were good and quasi-experiments were bad and could yield no useful information about program effectiveness. It is only in the past five to ten years that the notions of quasi-experimentation have been developed to the point where a sufficient intellectual rationale for their use exists (Cook and Campbell, 1979). There are, of course, problems associated with the use of such designs, but these are better dealt with in the context of a particular study than in terms of a general set of rules.

The single biggest obstacle to the use and, more important, the interpretation of results from quasi-experimental studies lies in estimating effects.

In a quasi-experimental study in which a comparison group is used (I personally avoid using the word "control" in connection with quasi-experimental studies since the term usually does not apply), estimates of program effects usually come from comparing the performance of the treatment group to that of a comparison group. Such a procedure presumes that the groups can indeed be compared. In quasi-experimental studies, it is necessary to build a case for basic comparability. Whether this can be done or not depends largely on the perspicacity of the investigator in the selection of the comparison group. If basic comparability can be established, then the investigator can use the comparative results to estimate program effects. The investigator would also be under heavy obligation to rule out each threat to internal validity on the grounds of evidence, experience, previous research, and logic. It can be done but it's not easy.

The current view with regard to the design and conduct of educational studies is that there is a large number of experimental and quasi-experimental designs available. Which one would be used in any particular study would depend more on local conditions than on the inherent characteristics of one design or another. The emphasis is clearly on selecting and adapting a design to meet local requirements. For example, if political, administrative or logistical factors prevent the use of randomization, then a quasi-experimental non-equivalent comparison group design might profitably be used. In the early stages of a program of continuing education, even a single-group pretest-treatment-posttest study might be profitably employed. If the content of the program is highly specialized and technical, even the use of such a quasi-experimental design could furnish an initial estimate of a program effect while also providing useful information about how the program might be strengthened. In short, the emphasis is on investigator inventiveness in thinking through a set of local conditions and deciding on a design that is best suited to those conditions. Threats to internal validity may have to be dealt with outside the framework of the design itself. As Cook and Campbell state,

> Estimating the internal validity of a relationship is a deductive process in which the investigator has to systematically think through how each of the internal validity threats may have influenced the data. Then the investigator has to examine the data to test which relevant threats can be ruled out. In all of this process, the researcher has to be his or her own best critic, trenchantly examining all of the threats he or she can imagine. When all of the threats can be plausibly eliminated, it is possible to make confident conclusions about whether a relationship is probably causal. When all of them cannot, perhaps because the appropriate data are not available or because the data indicate that a particular threat may indeed have operated, then the investigator has to conclude that a demonstrated relationship between two variables may or may not be causal. Sometimes

the alternative interpretations may seem implausible enough to be ignored and the investigator will be inclined to dismiss them. They can be dismissed with a special degree of confidence when the alternative interpretations seem unlikely on the basis of findings from a research tradition with a large number of relevant and replicated findings (Cook and Campbell, 1979, pp. 55-56).

Clearly, when randomization is possible, it should be used since it can be relied on to rule out most threats to internal validity and hence make causal inference easier. However, randomization is not a panacea. Randomization does not rule out all threats to internal validity. Diffusion or imitation of treatments and resentful demoralization, in particular, are not controlled through randomization and would hence need to be checked. More importantly, the extent of program executions is not assured through randomization. This is a critical point. Any study of program effectiveness is based on the assumption that the program has been carried out. It may or may not have been. In the field of education, two of the most famous studies of all time were fatally flawed by a failure to execute the program. The same could be true in the field of continuing education for the health professions where individuals did not faithfully complete programs of self-study or were frequently absent from sited programs. It is vital that in any study of program effects, efforts must be made to determine the extent to which a program was carried out and that participants who were supposed to receive the educational treatment actually did.

External Validity

Internal validity, as noted earlier, is concerned with the establishment of causal differences. External validity, on the other hand, is concerned with issues of generalizability. In an earlier era, McCall was suspicious of laboratory studies and questioned whether effects produced in laboratory settings would hold up in field settings. Since almost everyone was in a field setting, McCall forcefully argued for the conduct of studies in such settings. Campbell and Stanley (1963) took a similar position. This does not settle the issue of external validity, however.

The issue of external validity is highly complex and raises fundamental questions about the distinctions between research and evaluation. The research enterprise seeks to produce generalizable knowledge. When a chemist conducts an experiment to determine the coefficient of expansion of a particular metal under particular conditions of temperature and pressure, he is seeking to establish facts that will generalize broadly. The educational researcher strives for the same thing: generalizability. Under what conditions do particular kinds of people learn certain things? The research literature abounds with such studies, some good and, unfortunately, many bad.

The evaluation worker faces a different set of concerns. He or she is concerned with assessing the effectiveness of a particular program in a particular site with a particular group of learners and, if it's a didactic program, with particular instructors. There is little, if any, concern with whether the program would work elsewhere in the county, let alone another region of the country with different instructors, different learners and the like. The evaluation worker is typically so busy assessing the effects of the program in a single site or, at most, in a few carefully chosen ones, that there is little time to even consider issues of generalizability. And even if there were time for such musings, I suspect that the evaluation worker would rather quickly conclude that any attempts at generalizability are apt to be futile.

A program of continuing medical education is usually mounted to meet a particular need, often a local one. The people who develop the program and teach it are typically committed to it. Thus, instructor-effects are often confounded with treatments-effects, posing problems for the research worker but not for the evaluation worker. The researcher would like to obtain separate estimates of instructor- and program-effects. The evaluation worker, on the other hand, is concerned with establishing the combined effects of the two. The first order of business for the evaluation worker is to determine if the treatment (program *and* instructors) is producing real and meaningful effects. This is a big and important job. Once real and important program effects have been established and replicated with cohorts of learners *at the same site*, then one *might* turn one's attention to disentangling instructor- from program-effects and/or seek to establish the generalizability of the treatment in other places.

This rarely is done, however, and there are several reasons for it. Funding limitations often prevent such activities. Then, too, the magnitude of the effects is often not large enough to warrant exporting the program. Finally, the lack of control over what happens in a different setting is apt to make program developers and evaluation workers somewhat reluctant to export their wares. If the program does not produce the desired effects in a different setting, is it due to failures in program execution, instructor differences, learner differences — or something else? Such questions are largely unanswerable. They are troublesome ones for a researcher but less so for the evaluation worker whose assignment is to assess the total treatment effect in a single setting.

Perhaps the distinction between research and evaluation that has been drawn here is too fine. However, the intention has been to open the issue of generalizability and to suggest that different people can take different positions. When I work as an evaluation specialist, I am not concerned with the issue of generalizability. When I conduct research, I am. Ultimately, I feel that both evaluation workers and researchers are concerned with the production of useful and generalizable knowledge. However, the two roles occupy different points on the knowledge-production continuum. The evaluation worker is involved at the early stages and often participates in program development activities throughout formative evaluation work. The researcher enters somewhat later after the development of a promising product that needs full-blown testing. For the present, I think it is only necessary to acknowledge the issue of external validity and to recognize that it is not a high-priority concern for an evaluation worker.

Development, Demonstration, and Research

Just as evaluation workers and researchers play somewhat different roles in the knowledge-production process, evaluation activities undertaken at different points in that process will differ, too. The creation of an effective educational program, whether it be in continuing medical education or some other area, is a difficult and complex undertaking. For purposes of ease, the process has been broken into three phases although it needs to be recognized that they overlap considerably. These phases are development, demonstration, and research.

The *development* phase comes first. It may or not be based on, or include within it, some research activity. The goal of the development phase is to produce a program that is designed to have strong effects on participant learning. In developing the program, judgments have to be made as to what kind of learning is sought — knowledge acquisition, enhancement of skills and techniques, diagnostic strategies, etc. Content and learning activities then need to be selected or created and organized into a coherent program. This requires considerable effort. Program developers often perform this task in a rather haphazard way. While there is concern for what is likely to work or not, crucial judgments are often made on a highly subjective and impressionistic basis. This is not the best way to develop a program.

Evaluation workers can contribute significantly to program development by arranging for and conducting small trials of program segments (not the whole program) to obtain information as to how a segment works, i.e., what people learn from it, and how it is received. In design terms, this involves the use of a one-group pretest-posttest design, or even a one-group posttest design. Samples would be small, rarely involving more than a dozen people per segment and, in many cases, only three or four. Such activities typically come under the heading of formative evaluation and are characterized by a good deal of informality. This is perfectly proper since the goal is not to test the program formally but to provide an evidential basis for making judgments to guide the development of the program. If more activity of this type were undertaken at the development stage, programs with stronger effects might result.

Another notable contribution that an evaluation worker can make at this stage of program development is to serve as a reviewer and critic of a program. Program developers are often an enthusiastic group and tend to make claims for a program that cannot be realized. For example, a didactic program of continuing medical education may among its objectives have statements about increased ability to diagnose certain medical conditions but will not contain learning activities to develop such an ability. A knowledgeable evaluation worker can point these things out early on so that changes in the objectives, the learning activities, or both can be made.

An evaluation worker is often responsible for the development of instruments for assessing participant learning in terms of the program's objectives. Such work should commence in the development stage. The informal tryouts of program segments also affords an opportunity, albeit limited, for testing out instruments. More important, however, is the task of relating instruments to both objectives and learning activities so that objectives, learning activities and instruments form a coherent entity. Such matters can hardly be taken for granted.

It is not possible to say how long the period of development will last. Indeed, it may never end. At some point, however, the developers will want to try out the program as a whole under conditions of intended use. This is usually called a field trial or demonstration. At this point, the evaluation worker is usually expected to assume a major role in arranging and conducting the demonstration. Instruments for measuring program effects may be ready for use along with a number of supplemental measures. A comprehensive evaluation at this stage would include gathering the following kinds of information.

1. Initial status of learners
   a. descriptive information about learners — who they are and previous experience in area to be covered by program
   b. initial level of proficiency
2. Later status of learner — level of proficiency at completion of program
3. Execution of program — descriptive information about what took place in program, especially deviations from planned program
4. Supplemental information
   a. views/reactions/opinions of participants and instructors about program

b. supplemental learnings — learnings *not* covered by program objectives but considered part of the domain in which the program is based
c. side effects — unintended effects, either positive or negative, that can be attributed to the program. Usually detected through unstructured interviews and followup studies (adapted from Wolf, 1984, pp. 23–30).

Clearly, this is a tall order for any evaluation worker, requiring the use of a number of instruments as well as a set of associated studies (see 4c above). The goal of the evaluation activity is a rather fine-grained study of how the program is working and the effects it is having. If the demonstration phase involves the use of a control or comparison group, then the task will be even greater. Data analysis and interpretation will be formidable, but the payoffs should be enormous.

The results of the demonstration will usually lead to some further modifications in the program and, eventually, a large field trial. This is what the organizers of this conference term the research phase. It can also be called a field study or a large-scale field trial. The evaluation worker is needed to help plan and organize such an effort and often plays a central role in carrying it out. In this phase of work, the earlier distinction between evaluation and research becomes rather blurred. The goal here is to plan and conduct a true experiment or, at least, a quasi-experiment that will yield interpretable results. The design of such a study is unlikely to resemble one of the formal designs set forth in Campbell and Stanley (1963) or Cook and Campbell (1979) since it will undoubtedly contain a number of compromises between theoretical elegance and utter necessity. Since such a study will be considerably larger in scope than the demonstration, some sacrifices will have to be made. Usually, some aspects of the fine-grained data collection will have to be sacrificed because of practical constraints. However, the collection of pretest and posttest performance of participants in terms of the program's objectives is a *sine qua non* in the research phase. Any additional data that can be gathered without overburdening the resources of the project should be collected. Data analysis and interpretation of results will undoubtedly pose some problems, but these will be ably dealt with by Cooley.

Outcome Measures

The issue of outcome measures in programs in continuing medical education is, at once, quite straightforward and hideously complex. It is straightforward in the sense that a set of realistic program objectives and learning activities should provide a solid base for the creation and/or selection of outcome measures. Standard works on testing (Thorndike and Hagen, 1977, and Gronlund, 1981) furnish clear guidelines and offer specific procedures for the development of educational outcome measures. Thus, for example, if a program of continuing medical education is intended to increase physician knowledge on a particular topic, outcome measures for the program should seek to determine the knowledge state of the physician with regard to the topic that was studied.

That is not good enough, however. The presumption underlying continuing education is as follows:

Continuing Medical Education	Increased Physician Competence	Improved Physician Performance	Improved Patient Health Status
(A)	(B)	(C)	(D)

Continuing Medical Education (A) $\longrightarrow$ Increased Physician Competence (B) $\longrightarrow$ Improved Physician Performance (C) $\longrightarrow$ Improved Patient Health Status (D)

Each arrow in the above diagram denotes a causal link. The causal chain appears simple. In fact, some may feel it is simplistic. What is clearly missing from the causal chain are other variables that can influence the relationships between the variables listed. Being an outsider to the medical profession, I can only guess at what these might be. For example, besides Increased Physician Competence (B) influencing Improved Physician Performance (C), I can envisage that time and resources can also influence C. For example, if a physician is heavily burdened with patients, he or she may not have the time to do all the things that he or she would like to do. Also, if technical resources are lacking or in short supply, the physician may not be in a position to take a particular action that he or she would wish. Similarly, there can be intervening influences between A and B. A physician who is very busy may not be able to devote the time that is needed to a self-study program of continuing medical education and, consequently, does not show much of an increase in competence. Does one fault the program? I think not. Finally, the arrow between C and D suggests a strong link between the two. I do not readily accept this for two reasons. First, I do not believe that the state of medical knowledge is that complete or that certain. Second, I believe that here, too, there are other variables that can influence D besides C. I would put noncompliance by patients as a possible intervening variable here. Whether the tendency to practice defensive medicine comes between C and D or between B and C is unclear. I do believe that it should be put somewhere.

The model on which continuing medical education is based would appear to be too simplistic. Other factors are clearly involved. This does not mean that one should despair. The job is to get on with a program of research that seeks to identify and assess the factors that are involved. A series of small-scale studies can serve to help identify such factors. Until this can be done, one should probably restrict evaluation studies to assessing the *A-B* relationship in terms of limited and focused program objectives. To regard a continuing education as a failure because it does not bring about a change in patient health status is unduly harsh. It is quite plausible that the evaluation was a failure since it set unrealistic expectations.

A Final Note

The field of health care has had some great successes. We have miracle drugs and advanced surgical procedures that can bring dramatic results. In contrast, programs of continuing education must be regarded as weak treatments. Programs of self-study unloaded on often overworked practicing health-care professionals who are not in a position to give the time and effort required for mastery should not be expected to produce large effects. Until more powerful programs are developed, it would seem reasonable to adjust expectations to a more realistic level.

The future holds considerable promise for the field of continuing education for health-care professionals. Many of you can hasten its arrival by the work you do. Until then, the task in evaluation is to help set realistic expectations for programs in continuing education for health-care professionals, assess the extent to which they are being achieved, and in those cases where they are not being achieved, find out why not.

References

Campbell, D.T. and Stanley, J. (1963). "Experimental and quasi-experimental designs for research on teaching." In N.L. Gage (ed.), *Handbook of research on teaching*. Chicago: Rand McNally.

Cook, T.D. and Campbell, D.T. (1979). *Quasi-experimentation: Design and analysis issues for field settings*. Chicago: Rand McNally.

Gronlund, N. (1981). *Measurement and evaluation in teaching*. New York: Macmillan.

McCall, W.A. (1923). *How to experiment in education*. New York: Macmillan.

Thorndike, R.L. and Hagen, E.P. (1977). *Measurement and evaluation in psychology and education*. New York: John Wiley.

Wolf, R.M. (1984). *Evaluation in education*. 2nd edition. New York: Praeger.

5 CONTEMPORARY EVALUATION DESIGNS[1] IN CONTINUING EDUCATION

James T. Martinoff

During the past decade the desire to improve programs in continuing education for the health professions has witnessed the utilization of an increasing variety of evaluation designs. These variations have resulted from differences in the purpose, significance, and methodologies used in the conduct of program evaluations. It is the intent of this chapter to trace the evolution, and to identify and describe the principal types, of evaluation design currently being used in continuing education for the health professions.

Introduction

Prior to 1975, the practice of evaluation was little different from the practice of basic research. At that time, both research and evaluation had the same concern with internal validity and reliability, and for protecting the research environment from extraneous variables. Methodological rigor was the primary, often the only, criterion by which evaluation design was judged, including experimental designs (hypothesis testing under controlled conditions), quantitative data, multivariate, parametric statistical analysis, validation through replication, and external validity (Cronbach, 1975). However, rarely, if ever, were research designs effective in the evaluation of continuing education because the criteria of a "true experiment" could not be satisfied; the context of continuing education was not controlled; continuing education took place in "naturalistic" settings in a classroom, not in the laboratory (Hemphill, 1969). As a result, the research-design model was impractical because it interfered with the original purpose of the evaluation process which was to assist decision-makers in rendering judgment on the worth of a program (Worthen and Sanders, 1973).

In the last ten years, the practice of evaluation has changed considerably. The traditional emphasis placed on methodological rigor associated with research design has evolved into a more broad-based set of standards specifically concerned with the purpose, significance, and methodology of "evaluation design" (House, 1978). These standards recognize there is no one best way to conduct evaluations routinely; every evaluation is unique. As a result, the continuing-education evaluator must remain flexible and realistic about matching methods to the specific needs of the program and its clients. The essential guidelines are that an evaluation must possess utility, feasibility, propriety, and accuracy; i.e., it must be useful, practical, ethical, and valid for each particular evaluation (Joint Committee on Standards, 1981).

The evaluation design emerges from the special characteristics and conditions of a particular context in which judgment criteria are usually multiple and diverse depending on the hypotheses to be tested, the specific questions to be answered, or the general problems to be solved for the decision-maker. This emphasis has allowed for new and innovative methods to be used in evaluation design and is readily reflected in the current literature in the health professions (Bertram and Brooks-Bertram, 1977; Lloyd and Abrahamson, 1979; Stein, 1981).

The Classification System

To understand better the similarities and differences among the more than 100 different types of evaluation design that have been defined in the education literature (Patton, 1981) (and have subsequently been used in one form or another in the evaluation of programs in continuing education for the health professions), it was necessary to develop a simple but comprehensive classification system. The system was based upon consideration of the evaluation's purpose, significance, and methods. Evaluation purpose was principally concerned with the intent of the evaluation and the primary emphasis of the questions that were being asked. Evaluation significance was concerned with the role and relative importance of the evaluator and the intended use of the results. Evaluation methods were concerned with the systems utilized for the collection, analysis, and synthesis of data.

An integration of these three issues indicated the presence of three major categories or "types of evaluation activities" (Houle, 1980). Hoffman (1983) has defined these three categories as:

1. "Instructional Studies" which define evaluation as the process of determining whether or not educational objectives have been achieved;
2. "Inquiry Studies" which define evaluation as the process of providing information for decision-making; and
3. "Impact Studies" which define evaluation as the process of assessing the merit or worth of some object.

From these three categories of evaluation activity, four classes of evaluation design tend to dominate the evaluation systems utilized for the evaluation of continuing education in the health professions. These four classes of evaluation design include: Systems-Analysis Evaluation Design; Utilization-focused Evaluation Design; Professional Judgment Evaluation Design; and Goal-free Evaluation Design. A fifth evaluation design, Applied Research Evaluation Design, will be presented first, although its utility in the evaluation of continuing education has not been demonstrated.

Applied Research Evaluation Design

Building upon strong traditions from science, the purpose of Applied Research Evaluation Design has been to establish cause-and-effect relationships between continuing-education experiences and desired outcomes of the process (Stanley, 1972). Such an inquiry would require the use of control groups, valid data-collection systems, extensive followup procedures, as well as screening for extraneous variables, because continuing education does not characteristically take place over a sustained period of time within a reasonably controlled environment. It is a situation-specific process and its results cannot usually be generalized. While the potential of Applied Research Evaluation Design has been speculated by many (Riecken and Boruch, 1974; Rivlin and Timpane, 1975; Cook and Campbell, 1979), it has never been successfully implemented in the evaluation of continuing education for the health professions.

From an evaluation perspective, this design is based on a commonly recognized, though narrow, traditional view which simply equates evaluation with measurement and rejects the role of judgment by the evaluator. Evaluation here means to systematically measure results, effects, or performance, using some type of formalized objective instrument which produces data that can be compared to a standardized scale. In this design, the role of the evaluator is, of necessity, primarily that of an expert in the development and/or use of the measurement instruments that are to be employed, including an understanding of how results should be analyzed and presented. Communication between the evaluator and a "client" administrator is likely to be limited to a discussion of the measurement goal of testing for deterministic relationships. Feedback to the administrator will probably come in the nature of a formal report which may be limited to a simple display of the results of the application of the instrument. The expected outcome from the Applied Research Evaluation Design is a number or set of numbers which can be compared and interpreted with reference to another set of numbers, or generally accepted standard scale. The evaluator plays a passive role in decision-making and merely informs the administrator of the findings of the study, without becoming involved in the formulation of conclusions about the worth of the continuing-education activity. In this evaluation design, interpretation and judgment are the responsibility of the administrator.

Although this design implies that the test-and-measurement technology is highly complex and sophisticated, the methodology is conceptually quite simple. It usually consists of three components: *Inputs* (usually participant characteristics or attributes); the *Program* (those continuing-education experiences to which the participants are exposed); and *Outcomes* (certain targeted skills and abilities measured at program completion). Generally, participants are subjected to various program experiences and tested to determine whether participants in one group (program) exceeded, matched, or fell below those in another on some outcome measure. Program impact is inferred when outcome variance cannot be explained by input data alone, and when one group is significantly different from another. Where true experiments are not possible, quasi-experimental techniques, utilizing matrix sampling, are utilized to investigate cause-and-effect relationships between dependent (output) and independent (input) variables (Campbell and Stanley, 1963). For this design, since internal and external validity are the principal criteria, a comparison group is required if randomization of subjects to the educational treatment is not possible. Statistical techniques such as analysis of variance, analysis of covariance, and multiple analysis of variance are usually associated with this design.

In summary, Applied Research Evaluation Designs are used when high objectivity and reliability (comparability) are required, when relevant measurable attributes can be identified and valid intruments can be designed and implemented to measure them, and when mathematically manipulable results are desired for statistical analysis. As mentioned previously, this design, although frequently used, is hardly ever utilized in its entirety because the context of continuing education is almost always in a "naturalistic" (classroom) setting and neither it, nor its participants, can be controlled.

Systems Analysis Evaluation Design

Whereas Applied Research Evaluation Design attempts to understand cause-and-effect relationships within an environment by isolating the effects of a single variable, while holding all other factors constant, the Systems Analysis Evaluation Design is based on the assumption that there is no such thing as an "independent" variable; everything is ultimately related to everything else. In continuing education, this design considers all aspects of a program as being interrelated, and changes in any one particular component may have implications throughout the larger system. For example, earlier in this Conference, Wolf (1983) briefly outlined the assumptions that need to be tested in such a system that would relate to continuing education in the health professions:

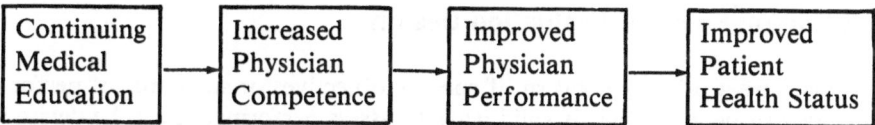

There are several articles in the literature which have used this evaluation design in attempting to assess the effect of continuing medical education on practice patterns and patient care (Talley, 1978; Wirtshafter et al. 1979; Pinkerton et al., 1980).

The purpose of this design is to identify the relationships among program components, between groups, and between the program and other larger systems. The primary emphasis of this type of evaluation design is on the program context and the environmental constraints, which may have an impact on the ultimate outcome of the program. In this design, the objectives are multiple, diverse, and long-term, and may or may not be interrelated. Some of the objectives may not become manifest until mid-way through the program, depending on changing conditions in the total educational environment.

At all times the evaluator is playing a very active role in determining how the program is interacting with the environment. A central position must be assumed, processing and integrating information from several sources. Much of the data that are collected in Systems Analysis Evaluation Designs also need to be interpreted since many of the data-collection techniques are nonquantitative in nature (Filstead, 1970). While this role in interpretation represents expansion in comparison with that in the Applied Research Evaluation Design, it is usually limited to data reduction and synthesis, rather than on extracting meaning as it relates to decisions affecting institutional policy. As a result, a continual exchange of information occurs between evaluators and "client" administrators as the program responds to and is affected by its environment, but final interpretation of the data is generally assumed to be the sole responsibility of the administrator.

The methodology for Systems Analysis Evaluation Design usually assumes predetermined objectives to be assessed, but is flexible enough to accommodate variables not predetermined. Although random assignment and control groups are desirable, they are not always possible, and quasi-experimental designs are found to be more realistic in this approach than true experiments. Multivariate techniques, trait-treatment interaction studies, correlational analysis, and nonquantitative procedures (Patton, 1980), such as exploratory data analysis, naturalistic inquiry, modeling, simulation, and a variety of other qualitative techniques, are examples of analyses that have been used in the evaluation of continuing-education programs.

Utilization-Focused Evaluation Design

If goals are a primary concern, if specific objectives or standards of performance can be identified, if valid ways to assess performance can be devised and applied, and if effects unrelated to stated goals are of little or no importance, then a Utilization-Focused Evaluation Design ought to be utilized. The principal emphasis of this design is to define which information is needed and wanted by decision-makers, information-users, and stakeholders, and that will actually be used for program improvement and to make decisions about the program (Patton, 1978). A major advantage of the Utilization-Focused Evaluation Design is that it requires continuing-education professionals to conceptualize and clearly articulate the objectives of the program and the goals of management. The desired outcome of this evaluation design is extended communication between evaluators and the client administrators regarding information needs associated with critical decisions. The three main elements of this approach are that relevant decision-makers and information-users must be identified and organized; evaluators must work actively and flexibly with the information-users and stakeholders to make decisions about the evaluation focus and methods; and all individuals involved in the evaluation design must continually ask the question, "What would you do with this information?" This design emphasizes pragmatism and utility. Perhaps no other type of evaluation in recent continuing-education literature has received more attention in determining whether a program or activity should be maintained, improved, expanded, or terminated (R.M. Caplan, personal communication).

The implied role of the evaluator in this design is to assist program management and to serve the decision-maker. Because the objectives of the program are clearly articulated and accepted as a part of the project design and judgment criteria are pre-established by the objectives, little opportunity is left for the evaluator to determine the appropriateness of the objective themselves. As a result of the emphasis on specific, short-term, measurable objectives, the evaluator must make certain that longer-term, higher-order objectives, effects of which cannot be expected to fully accrue during the program, are still considered an important outcome of the program (Cooley and Lohnes, 1978). This has specific implications for continuing education because all too often only cognitive objectives that are easily measured are defined, and other objectives in the affective domain which may be equally important are treated as intangible and relatively unimportant because of their difficulty in measurement. This fact is made very clear in Stoeckle's (1979) work on humanistic dimensions of medical education.

Therefore, it is the role of the evaluator to consult continually with information-users and decision-makers to see that multiple objectives from all three domains of behavior are included in the evaluation design, even though their primary role is simply to compare outcomes with stated objectives, and report differences between expected and actual results to decision-makers, who have the responsibility to act accordingly. Scriven confirms that in a formative evaluation (process-oriented evaluation used to improve an ongoing project by providing feedback), the evaluator should be prepared not only to clarify and identify new objectives through needs analysis (Kaufman, 1977) but also to make an assessment of the worth of the objectives themselves (Scriven, 1974). Others carry this a step further by suggesting that expert evaluators should be involved from the beginning of any program or project, and should be instrumental in defining its objectives and the feasibility of collecting relevant performance data (Suchman, 1970; Stufflebeam et al., 1971). Where a summative (end-product-oriented) evaluation is desired, the evaluator's primary function will most likely be an after-the-fact determination of the previously defined goals of the project through interaction with participants and a review of documentation.

The evaluator must also be expert in measurement methodology relative to the concept of program to be evaluated, as well as in the collection and analysis of performance data. The judgments of program worth may be made by the evaluator or by the administrator based on the information supplied by the evaluator. This interpretation is based on the relative discrepancy on congruence between objectives and results (Provus, 1973).

The methodology for this design is similar to that of Management Information Systems designed to provide information for project, program, and system decisions. The three major areas of the methodology include focusing the evaluation (i.e., identifying the specific decision situations to be served, and defining the criteria to be used in the judgment of alternatives) and collecting, organizing, analyzing, and reporting information. As with previous designs, quasi-experimental designs appear to be more appropriate because of the difficulty of random assignment and control groups.

Professional Judgment Evaluation Design

In situations where a high degree of objectivity is not required, where time is short, where a relatively simple evaluation approach is desired, and expert human resources are available, the Professional Judgment Evaluation Design (or Panel of Experts Evaluation Design) may be most appropriate. The utility of this relatively informal evaluation design is evidenced in the numerous situations where a qualified professional or group of professionals is asked to examine a continuing-education program, and then to render an expert opinion regarding its quality, effectiveness, or efficiency. The primary focus of this design is that the best judge of worth is an expert in the area to be evaluated.

The role of the evaluator, thus, is quite different from that in the earlier designs. The role is that of an information-processor whose job is to assimilate and judge relevant information. Skill in synthesizing and weighing facts is assumed, in addition to expertise in the domain or activity to be evaluated.

The methodology of this design provides for personal contact between the evaluator and the program or activity to be evaluated. The outcome may be of little personal concern if the evaluator is an outsider called in to evaluate some aspect of a program. In such a case, the values brought to bear might be said to be relatively objective. On the other hand, if the evaluator has a personal stake in the process, as, for example, in the case of evaluating the teaching effectiveness of a fellow faculty member, the needs of the department, college, and personalities will probably have a bearing on the evaluation process.

The particular methods used in the Professional Judgment Evaluation Design may include personal observation, interviews, testing, review of documentation, etc. — in short, whatever kind of experiential contact is deemed necessary and agrees with client administrator expectations. However, the assimilation of the data collected is internal; that is, the final report, whether formal or informal, emanates from the evaluators' thought processes. The desired outcome is the educated opinion of the evaluator; his or her interpretation is generally expressed in the form of a pronouncement. It is in this evaluation design that the evaluator assumes the most powerful role, even though his pronouncements are either accepted or rejected by the administrator at his or her prerogative.

Examples of this type of evaluation design include reliance on the judgments of a director of continuing education on whether particular courses ought to be taught, who will teach them, and/or when they will be offered. "Panel-of-Experts Evaluation Design," which may also fall under this classification of "professional judgment," is associated with the use of (1) peer-review panels to evaluate teaching effectiveness, (2) visitation teams of professionals sent by the various accrediting associations (although these are usually based on a comprehensive self-study and set of objectives), (3) the use of expert referees in the process of selecting manuscripts for publication, and (4) the passing of judgment on the candidates for promotion or tenure by faculty committees.

Goal-Free Evaluation Design

If all observable effects are potentially relevant, if human concerns are uppermost, if a relatively high degree of objectivity is not required, and if the situation is highly fluid and lacking well-defined goals and/or traditional measurement data, a Goal-Free (Scriven, 1973) or Responsive Evaluation Design (Stake, 1975) may be the most appropriate. This design begins with the premise that evaluators seldom are aware of all of the criteria upon which they or others will make a judgment of program merit. The intent of this design is to discover and judge actual effects without regard to what the effects were supposed to be. Scriven has argued that if the main objective of the evaluation is to assess the worth of outcomes, why make any distinction between those that were intended, as opposed to those that were not? What is proposed in Goal-Free Evaluation Design is allowing the evaluator to select wider-context goals as opposed to only those prespecified in mission statements, objectives, or program design. In this design, the evaluator is seen as an investigator skilled in identifying important relationships and outcomes.

The role of the evaluator who uses this evaluation design is to operate informally, though systematically, in an environment of continual interaction with others, drawing conclusions and descriptive information out of the observations and reactions of the persons involved. This requires that the evaluator be skilled in social interaction, in eliciting honest comments and opinions, and in capturing and recording conversations (Smith, 1982). Interpretation of the results by the evaluator should be responsive to the concerns of the individuals affected, whether they are program participants or those who commissioned the study.

The methodology of this design acquires information about a program through an iterative process, defining the issues of importance to constituencies, and describing the strengths and weaknesses relative to those issues. In this design, meaningful data are possible only through in-depth description of the program in context and through the personal testimony of participants (Friedlander, 1982). Stated objectives may or may not be centrally important to the issues identified as a result of the iterative process. In this design, all issues of interest to the constituents are taken into consideration initially, but no single element is preconceived as being necessarily more important to the evaluator than another. Variables are not preselected but emerge in the process of describing the operation of the program in its naturalistic setting. This evaluation design neither controls nor ignores internal and external pressures, but takes great effort in describing them. Eisner (1979) feels that phenomenologically based information has greater validity than data obtained from traditional, structured, measurement instruments. As a result of this approach, experimental designs are rejected as inappropriate for understanding socially imbedded programs and their effects on participants (Guba, 1978).

Note

1. The concept of evaluation design can be construed as the skeletal framework or organizational model which, like a blueprint, sets the foundation for observation and measurement. This term refers to the designated system for the definition, collection, and analysis of data that assess the effectiveness of a given program. Its purpose is to plan, organize, direct, and control the evaluation procedure. The product of this process is to assist decision-makers responsible for deciding policy in rendering judgment on the worth of a program or activity.

For purposes of this chapter, no distinctions are made between evaluation design and the following concepts: evaluation framework, evaluation model, evaluation system, and evaluation approach.

References

Bertram, D.A. and Brooks-Bertram, P.A. (1977). "The evaluation of continuing medical education: A literature review." *Health Education Monographs*, 5, 330–348.

Campbell, D.T. and Stanley, J. (1963). "Experimental and quasi-experimental designs for research on teaching." In N.L. Gage (ed.), *Handbook of research on teaching.* Chicago: Rand McNally.

Cook, T.D. and Campbell, D.T. (1979). *Quasi-experimentation: Design and analysis issues for field settings.* Chicago: Rand McNally.

Cooley, W.W. and Lohnes, P.R. (1976). *Evaluation research in education.* New York: Irvington Publishers.

Cronbach, L.J. (1975). "Beyond the two disciplines of scientific psychology." *American Psychologist,* 30, 116–127.

Eisner, E.W. (1979). "The use of qualitative forms of evaluation for improving educational practice." *Educational Evaluation and Policy Analysis,* 1(6), 11–19.

Filstead, W.J. (ed.). (1970). *Qualitative methodology.* Chicago: Markham.

Friedlander, F. (1982). "Alternative modes of inquiry." *Small Group Behavior,* 13, 428–440.

Guba, E.G. (1978). *Toward a methodology of naturalistic inquiry in educational evaluation.* Los Angeles: UCLA Center for the Study of Evaluation.

Hemphill, J.K. (1969). "The relationship between research and evaluation studies." In R.W. Tyler (ed.), *Educational evaluation: New roles, new means.* Sixty-eighth Yearbook of the National Society for the Study of Evaluation. Chicago: University of Chicago Press, pp. 189–220.

Hoffman, K.I. (1983). *Recapitulation: Another view of data analysis.* Paper presented at the Conference on Evaluation of Continuing Education in the Health Professions: State of the Art, University of Southern California, Los Angeles.

Houle, C.O. (1980). *Continuing learning in the professions.* San Francisco: Jossey-Bass.

House, E.R. (1978). "Assumptions underlying evaluation models." *Educational Researcher,* 7(3), 4–12.

Joint Committee on Standards for Educational Evaluation. (1981). *Standards for evaluation of educational programs, projects, and materials.* New York: McGraw-Hill.

Kaufman, R. (1977). "A possible taxonomy of needs assessment." *Educational Technology,* 17(11), 60–64.

Lloyd, J.S. and Abrahamson, S. (1979). "Effectiveness of continuing medical education: A review of the evidence." *Education and the Health Professions,* 2(3), 251–280.

Patton, M.Q. (1978). *Utilization-focused evaluation.* Beverly Hills: Sage Publications.

Patton, M.Q. (1980). *Qualitative evaluation methods.* Beverly Hills: Sage Publications.

Patton, M.Q. (1981). *Creative evaluation.* Beverly Hills: Sage Publications.

Pinkerton, R.E., Tinaoff, N., Willms, J.L., and Tapp, J.T. (1980). "Resident physician performance in a continuing education format: Does newly acquired knowledge improve patient care?" *Journal of the American Medical Association,* 244(19), 2183–2185.

Provus, M. (1973). *Discrepancy evaluation.* Berkeley: McCutchan Publishing.

Riecken, H.W., and Boruch, R.F. (1974). *Social experimentation: A method for planning and evaluating social intervention.* New York: Academic Press.

Rivlin, A.M. and Timpane, T.M. (eds.). (1975). *Planned variation in education: Should we give up or try harder?* Washington, D.C.: Brookings Institute.

Scriven, M. (1973). "Goal-free evaluation." In E.R. House (ed.), *School evaluation: The politics and process.* Berkeley: McCutchan Publishing.

Scriven, M. (1974). "The concept of evaluation." In M. Apple, M. Subkoviak, and H. Lufler Jr. (eds.), *Educational evaluation: Analysis and responsibility.* Berkeley: McCutchan Publishing.

Smith, N.L. (1982). *Communication strategies in evaluation.* Beverly Hills: Sage Publications.

Stake, R.E. (Ed.). (1975). *Evaluating the arts in education: A responsive approach.* Columbus, Ohio: Merrill.

Stanley, J.C. (1972). "Controlled field experiments as a model for evaluation." In P.H. Rossi and W. Williams (eds.), *Evaluating social programs: Theory, practice, and politics.* New York: Seminar Press, pp. 67–71.

Stein, L.S. (1981). "The effectiveness of continuing medical education: A research report." *Journal of Medical Education,* 56, 103–110.

Stoeckle, J.D. (1979). "The tasks of care: Humanistic dimensions of medical education." In W.R. Rogers and D. Bernard (eds.), *Nourishing the humanistic in medicine.* Pittsburgh: University of Pittsburgh Press.

Stufflebeam, D.L., Foley, W.J., Gephart, W.J., Guva, E.G., Hammond, H.D., Merriman, H.O., and Provus, N.M. (1971). *Educational evaluation and decision making.* Itasca, Illinois: F.E. Peacock.

Suchman, E.A. (1970). "The role of evaluative research." *Proceedings of the 1969 Invitational Conference on Testing Problems.* Princeton, New Jersey: Educational Testing Service, pp. 93–103.

Talley, R.C. (1978). "Effect of continuing medical education on practice patterns." *Journal of Medical Education,* 53(7), 602–603.

Wirtschafter, D.D., Sumners, J., Colvin, E., Knox, E., Turner, M., Cassady, G., Beale, P., Budrich, M., and Brooks, C.M. (1979). "Continuing medical education: An assessment of impact on neonatal care in community hospitals." *Proceedings of the 18th Annual Conference on Research in Medical Education.* Washington, D.C.: Association of American Medical Colleges, pp. 252–257.

Wolf, R.M. (1983). *Design Problems in evaluation.* Paper presented at the Conference on Evaluation of Continuing Education in the Health Professions: State of the Art, University of Southern California, Los Angeles.

Worthen, B.R. and Sanders, J.R. (eds.). (1973). *Educational evaluation: Theory and practice.* Worthington, Ohio: Charles A. Jones.

6 DATA-COLLECTION PROBLEMS IN EVALUATION

George F. Madaus

Introduction

When all three partners of the newly formed evaluation firm of DATAFAX, INC., were interviewed for a potential contract by the project directors, the company philosophy soon became clear: data and facts were the same thing — and the only thing. The junior partner, Joe Friday, when asked how they would proceed if awarded the contract replied, "All we want are the facts, ma'am."[1] When the project director inquired about a theoretical base for the evaluation, the second partner, Sherlock Holmes, immediately cautioned, "It is a capital mistake to theorize before one has data. Insensibly one begins to twist facts to suit theories instead of theories to suit facts" (Doyle, 1981, p. 163). Lest Holmes, the most erudite of the partners, be misunderstood, the senior partner and founder of the firm, Thomas Gradgrind, of Dickens fame, reminded the clients, "In this life, we want nothing but Facts, sir; nothing but Facts!" (1981, p. 25).

After being bombarded with this great positivistic gospel, the clients awarded the contract to DATAFAX, INC. Because, after all, with but a glance at the dictionary, the client confirmed that a fact is something known with certainty, something having real, demonstrable existence. It is perceived as real, solid, hard, irrefutable, substantive, true, and self-validating.

Naturally the clients believed that the foundation of an evaluation rests on the proposition that a fact is a fact. The necessary correlate of that proposition is, a fact is either right or wrong, which in turn implies that "the standard against which the rightness or wrongness of a fact may be judged exists someplace — perhaps graven upon a tablet in a Platonic world outside and above *this* cave of tears" (Perry, 1967, p. 23).

Even a moment's reflection, however, reveals that one person's "facts" are another's mere "opinion," "supposition," or worse still, "fiction." Thus what constitutes a fact often depends on the evaluator's or client's frame of reference. A fact in the last analysis is "an observation or an operation performed in a frame of reference" (Perry, 1967, p. 23). Maybe the medieval schoolmen were wise in enumerating the principle "Quid, quid recipitur per modum recipientis recipitur."[2]

In this chapter I shall do three things. First I shall point out problems associated with data collection, or fact-gathering, that relate to the evaluator's frame of reference. Second, I shall consider data collection from the point of view of the different roles associated with evaluation. And finally I shall consider data collection in terms of the Joint Committee on *Standards for Educational Evaluation*, in particular the 16 standards that directly relate to data collection. Throughout I shall refer to the "Heartmobile Proposal" and to the articles on the evaluation of continuing medical education (CME) that were part of the packets sent in advance of the Conference.

Part I: Data Collection and the Evaluator's Frame of Reference

The immunologist Peter Medawar (1982), in attempting to answer the question, "What is science?," describes two conceptualizations:

> . . . the romantic and the rational, or the "poetic" — in Shelley's sense ("poetry comprehends all science") — and the analytical, the one speaking for the imaginative insight and the other for the evidence of the senses. . . .

Similarly, there are two conceptions of evaluation, characterized by polar groups: the more traditional positivistic/quantitative evaluators at one pole and the recently emerging phenomenological/qualitative evaluators at the other (Madaus and McDonagh, 1982). While there are values and strengths associated with both of these conceptualizations, and while each can learn from the other, nonetheless, data collection and methods of evaluation are influenced by the evaluator's frame of reference, his/her world view and philosophy of evaluation.

Cronbach (1982) recognizes this dichotomy in the field when he contrasts a "scientistic" school of evaluation with a "humanistic" one. The former prize experiments; the latter find them misinformative. However, the differences go beyond arguments over the value of experimentation. The gap between the two cultures is wider and more profound, an embodiment of the doubts about the scientific method which the biologist Thomas (1979) describes in one of his marvelous books, *The Medusa and the Snail:*

> Science gets most of its information by the process of reductionism, exploring the details, of the details, until the smallest bits of the structure, or the smallest parts of the mechanism, are laid out for counting and scrutiny. Only when this is done can the investigation be extended to encompass the whole organism or the entire system. So we say . . . Sometimes it seems that we take a loss, working this way. Much of today's public anxiety about science is the apprehension that we may forever be overlooking the whole by an endless, obsessive preoccupation with the parts (p. 6).

The positivistic/quantitative evaluators tend toward the reductionism and quantitative emphasis described by Thomas. From their viewpiont, data are pieces of information or facts that have been put in numerical form.

The phenomenological/qualitative approach, typified by Guba's "naturalistic inquiry," Eisner's "connoisseurship evaluation," Stake's "responsive evaluation," Partlett and Hamilton's "illuminative evaluation," and Denny's case study or "story telling" approach, argue against the reductionism of the scientific approach. In their view the whole is equal to more than the sum of its parts. An evaluation should help the client and key publics to better understand the program. Data encompass a different order of facts from the numerical indices of the quantitative approach: data come from human observation, testimony, anecdotal evidence, and, most importantly, that gift that every good physician possesses, intuition. Often they use impressionistic techniques like those of Dickens in *Hard Times* where he was "concerned with factual material that would give the 'feel' of a system as well as a sense of the physical atmosphere in which it existed" (Spector, 1981, p. 15). The process for these evaluators is often as lyrical as it is empirical.

When I read works from the two approaches or, more compelling yet, when I teach about them as part of a course on evaluation models, I am reminded of C.P. Snow's (1962) observation.

> I felt I was moving among two groups — comparable in intelligence, identical in race, not grossly different in social origin, earning about the same incomes, who had almost ceased to communicate at all, who in intellectual, moral and psychological climate had so little in common that instead of going from Burlington House or South Kensington to Chelsea, one might have crossed an ocean (p. 2). . . . Their attributes are so different that even, on the level of emotion, they can't find much common ground (p. 4).

The differences in the way evaluation is conceptualized are much more than simply methodological differences about what data should be collected and how, or whether to conduct an experiment or not; they reflect basic ideological differences that underpin the respective approaches. In turn, these ideological differences between the two "cultures" are related in part to the respective training the evaluators received and in important part to differences in personality and temperament. Let us consider first the issue of training.

When the need for evaluations first began to emerge strongly during the '60s and then exploded in the early '70s, early practitioners of the evaluation art came out of a testing and research background. As was the case in sociology and psychology during the '30s, '40s, and '50s, there was a very strong temptation for practitioners in educational testing and research to adopt the natural science frame of reference in order to gain scientific acceptability. As a result, many practitioners tried to imitate what they wrongly believed to be the following three characteristics of the natural sciences: (1) the belief that measurement and numeration are intrinsically praiseworthy activities (the worship, indeed, of what Ernest Gambrich calls *idola quantitatis*); (2) the whole discredited farrago of inductivism — especially the belief that facts are prior to ideas and that sufficiently voluminous compilation of facts can be processed by a calculus of discovery in such a way as to yield general principles and natural-seeming laws; (3) . . . faith in the efficacy of statistical formulae, particulary when processed by a computer — the use of which is in itself interpreted as a mark of scientific manhood (Medawar, 1980, p. 167).

Thus, many of the early evaluators quite naturally applied their "scientific" tools of testing and research to problems of evaluating educational programs. As time passed, however, a growing dissatisfaction with the results of such evaluations, both on the part of clients and the evaluators themselves, prompted one of two reactions. The first was a call for more rigorous control, for better cooperation on the part of clients in the application of the scientific paradigm. The second was a disillusionment with the "scientific" method and a search for models of inquiry that might be better suited to addressing the problems confronted in an evaluation. Related to this reaction was the realization that interpersonal skills — skills not ordinarily taught as part of traditional graduate training in testing and research — were at least as important as any of the methodological skills that are taught. This second reaction on the part of many trained in the more traditional manner took the form, almost, of religious conversion, as these evaluators began to step to different drummers. Both reactions, it should be noted, were a sign of the emerging maturity of the field.

Today's evaluators are still being trained primarily in the tools of one culture or the other, although there is much more cross-fertilization than before, more awareness of other views, more communication between the camps than before. Nonetheless, programs that train evaluators tend to emphasize one approach over the other, and students internalize that approach which, subtly and not so subtly, affects how they approach evaluations and data collection.

But more than training is at issue. The representatives of the two cultures differ in temperament, inclination, and personality, and these affective differences influence greatly how they view evaluation and how they define, and go about collecting, data. As Medawar (1982) has pointed out, the distinctions between the two types of science, or in our case between the two types of evaluation, "do not hang together logically or rationally in themselves; rather they are complexes of opinion that tend to go with certain temperaments, much as Tory and Labour or Republican and Democrat stand for casts of thought as much as for casts of vote" (p. 13). These affective or temperamental differences also contribute to the lack of dialogue between some traditional evaluators and their naturalistic counterparts (Madaus and McDonagh, 1982).

Differences in training and personality affect data collection and lead the evaluator to construe reality as "fact" in a way quite different from reality by another evaluator. The following anecdote by A.L. Lloyd (1967) from the field of folk music beautifully illustrates the influence of training and temperament on how perception defines reality.

> One afternoon in a sombre room of the Ethnographical Museum in Budapest a well-known folklorist, colleague of Bartok and Kodaly, played his visitor a recording of a Casango-Magyar ballad singer from Moldavia. Her song was tragic and she performed it with a fine contained passion, in a way that showed she was totally immersed in the sense of the song. The visitor remarked on the poignant quality of the rendition and the learned professor gave him a sharp look and said: 'Surely by now you know that the sound of folk music is meaningless? It's not until we have it down in precise notation and can see what's happening inside the mould of the melody that it comes to have any significance at all.' For him, what the song meant to the singer was irrelevant; that it brought her almost to tears was a detail not worth inquiring into; the woman was a mere accessory and her heart, mind, voice were superfluities, unnecessary to take into account; pitch and duration were all that mattered. He was a good man for Kelvin's principle: What we measure can be understood (p. 17).

Like Lloyd's two musicologists, the evaluator brings the totality of personal history and background specialization to his/her work.[3]

What does all this mean in a CME evaluation? First, in hiring an evaluator the client should be acquainted with the prospective evaluator's frame of reference since it will affect the type of data that are eventually collected. Looking, for example, at the article in the *New England Journal of Medicine* by Sibley and associates (1980) as well as at the review by Lloyd and Abrahamson (1977) on the effectiveness of CME, it would appear that CME evaluations have been carried out within the traditional, positivistic/quantitative approach; that such an approach has been adopted is not surprising, given the nature of medical training and research and their roots in the natural sciences. The articles emphasize pretest, posttest designs, control groups, and traditional indicators of physician competence, physician performance, and improved patient health status. It may be that evaluations of CME have been pursuing an incorrect course with the maximum of precision (Deutscher, 1976). To turn the old saw, the operation was a success but CME died.

Second, and closely related, the person commissioning a CME evaluation needs to examine how his/her world view may be affecting the choice of one particular kind of evaluator over another. Deutscher (1976), while writing about another discipline, sociology, sums up the consequences of the choice of the positivistic approach to a CME evaluation.

> In attempting to assume the stance of physical science, we have necessarily assumed its epistemology — its assumptions about the nature of knowledge and the appropriate means of knowing, including the rules of scientific evidence. The requirement of clean empirical demonstration of the effects of isolated factors or variables, in a manner which can be replicated, led us to create, by definition, such factors or variables. We knew that human behavior was rarely if ever directly influenced or explained by an isolated variable; we knew that it was impossible to assume that any set of such variables was additive (with or without weighting); we knew that the complex mathematics of the interaction among any set of variables, much less their interaction with external variables, was incomprehensible to us. In effect, although we knew they did not exist, we defined them into being.

> But it was not enough just to create sets of variables. They had to be stripped of what little meaning they had in order that they might be operational, i.e., that they have their measurement built into their definition. One consequence, then, was to break down human behavior in a way that was not only artificial but which did not jibe with the manner in which that behavior was observed (p. 32–33).

It may be the time for those who commission evaluations of CME programs to take a more critical look at alternative approaches to evaluation which to date seem to have been neglected. They need to re-evaluate the consequences of their choices of a particular kind of evaluator.

Finally, a mix of approach should result in a more useful and more valid evaluation with different types of evaluators working as a team or independently, gathering quantitative and qualitative data, using traditional and human instrumentation. Of course this adds to the cost of the evaluation. Certainly an evaluation budget of $20,000 for an evaluator, only $5,000 more than the amount budgeted for a secretary and $40,000 less than the amount allocated for the project director, would not allow for much in the way of a multidisciplined approach.

Part II: The Roles of Evaluation and Data Collection

The type of question the evaluator is asked immediately focuses the task of data collection. While different evaluators may see the task of data collection differently, once the evaluator's role relative to a particular project has been defined, the nature of the data needed and how they can be collected have been narrowed considerably. For any given project, an evaluator can be asked to gather data to answer quite different types of questions.

In an attempt to focus the different types of questions evaluators are asked, I have taken Scriven's (1973) distinctions between evaluation questions that are formative and summative in nature and crossed them with Stufflebeam's (1973) four types of evaluation — context, input, process, and product — which correspond to four types of administrative decisions (planning, structuring, implementing, recycling). There is one addition. I have further partitioned the product cell of the matrix by using Scriven's (1973) distinction between "intrinsic" or secondary evaluation and "pay-off" or primary evaluation (see table 6-1).

A quick definition of the terms borrowed from Scriven may be in order before proceeding. *Formative evaluation* is geared to answering questions during the development stage of the project, and is generally carried out by an evaluator working directly for the project. The end of formative evaluation is to improve the project, or product, while it is still under development.

Table 6-1. Role of Evaluator and Type of Decision Served by Data Collection

	Context Evaluation (Planning Decisions)	Input Evaluation (Structuring Decisions)	Process Evaluation (Implementing Decisions)	Product Evaluation (Recycling Decisions) Intrinsic	Payoff
Formative	1	2	3	4	5
Summative	6	7	8	9	10

Summative evaluation, on the other hand, is generally done by an evaluator external to the project. It takes place after the project or product has been finalized. The end of summative evaluation is to answer questions about the adoption, recycling, or discontinuation of a program or product.

Intrinsic or secondary evaluation involves an appraisal of the project or product *itself.* It is concerned with the goals and procedures of the program, and with opinions about the program or product. Primary or payoff evaluation, on the other hand, looks at the *direct* effects of the program or product on the recipient and other concerned publics and at these alone. The Stufflebeam categories are self-explanatory.

Cell 1: Formative Context Evaluation

At the very beginning of the project the evaluator helps the client to define the social, political, and economic contexts in which the program will operate. Descriptive, demographic data can be gathered on characteristics of the population to be served, the community, the agency sponsoring and implementing the project, and/or other concerned publics and institutions. Appropriate techniques include surveys, examination of logs, records, newspaper clippings, legislative bills, demographic studies, and census data.

Another role for the evaluator in this cell of the matrix may be to conduct a needs assessment. Needs are assessed and opportunities are examined through an examination of census data, medical records, test scores, interviews, hearings, and social indicators of various kinds.[4]

Finally it is in this cell that the goals of a program themselves are evaluated. Too often, program goals have been accepted without evaluation of their reasonableness or their usefulness in meeting a need.

Cell 2: Formative Input Evaluation

Once the goals of the program have been evaluated and accepted, the evaluator can assist in identifying and assessing the available funds, resources, materials, facilities, staff, and staff training necessary to implement the goals. The evaluator gathers data to answer the question, "Are there disparities between goals and resources?" Formative input evaluation allows the staff to assess design implementation strategies while they are still flexible. Stufflebeam (1983) suggests that to answer these questions data can be collected, using such techniques as literature searches, visits to similar programs, pilot trials, and advocate team hearings.

The importance of the evaluator's role in this stage of project development would never be recognized from the number of times they are actually involved in this crucial early stage.

Cell 3: Formative Process Evaluation

Here the evaluator provides the staff with feedback on implementation, while the process still can be modified and improved. Implementation strategies are pretested to answer such questions as these. Can the teachers handle the material? How much variation in delivery is there from teacher to teacher and how much variation is appropriate? Do the recipients understand the instruction? Is the reading level of the material appropriate for the recipients? Are the target groups being reached? These developmental questions can be answered through data collected by direct observation, interviews, questionnaires, and expert analyses.

Cell 4: Formative Secondary Product Evaluation

Here the evaluator provides the developer with data about the product or treatment itself, while it is still under development. Some of the questions posed here overlap with questions in other cells (e.g., are the goals and objectives appropriate; is the readability level of material suitable?) Pilot-testing and pretesting of material would be designed to answer such questions as these. Is the content appropriate, interesting, challenging? Are the scope and sequence of content and objectives appropriate? Do teachers like the materials? Do students have mastery of the necessary enabling objectives? Do recipients like the material or instruction? Is it easy to administer?

These and similar questions can be answered by data collected through expert analyses and through observation, interviews, and questionnaires.

Cell 5: Formative Primary Product Evaluation

During the pretest phase, the evaluator provides feedback to the staff on how well recipients are achieving the intended objectives of each unit and feedback on any unintended outcomes — positive and negative. Keeping in mind that the data are meant to help the developer improve the program while it is still under development, the use of small samples and "quick-and-dirty" techniques of data collection are adequate here particularly during the pilot-testing phase. In fact, such techniques may be all that the evaluator can reasonably do, given the need for rapid feedback. Quick quizzes, direct questions, observations, examination of student products — these may be the most efficient techniques of data collection during development. Better developed pretests and posttests and other more structured techniques may be employed when the program is pretested. But even here the pretest may also be a tryout phase for these data-collection techniques themselves.

Cell 6: Summative Context Evaluation

This cell comprises an important, but sometimes neglected, aspect of program evaluation. Very often programs, particularly innovative ones, are funded because of perceived problems, not with the clients of an institution (e.g., students, patients, welfare recipients) but with the institution itself (e.g., schools, hospitals, social agencies). The object of funding programs in such cases is to install a demonstration program that will be so effective that the institution will be shamed into adopting it, thereby changing the institution for the better. Unfortunately, however, the evaluation of such efforts often focuses exclusively on the effects of the program on the recipients, or agency clients, rather than on the more difficult and politically sensitive issues of the changes brought about by the program on the institution per se.

Once the program has been implemented and has had a fair trial, the evaluator can assist the sponsoring agency in assessing the degree to which the program has altered the target institution. Has the operating context changed? Instead of assimilating the program has the institution coopted it through subtle and not-so-subtle modifications or omissions? Has the program met the needs identified in cell 1 of our matrix? Data collection in aid of these questions can include a pre- and postorganizational analysis through interviews, surveys, and client observation, and through the examination of documents, records, newspaper clippings, and of budgets and staffing patterns.

Cell 7: Summative Input Evaluation

Here the summative evaluator assists the client in determining the degree to which the resources allocated in the implementation strategy (cell 2) actually were delivered to the target groups as planned. Further, a key evaluation question included in this cell, but closely related to the summative primary product cell (cell 10), is whether or not the program is cost-effective. How does this program compare with others in terms of the money spent? What part of the money went to salaries; what part to services? What is the per-person cost of the program? (Fink and Kosecoff, 1983). Data to answer these questions can be collected through document and budget analyses, interviews, and observations. Levin (1974) describes a useful worksheet to help estimate program costs.

Cell 8: Summative Process Evaluation

Here the evaluator helps the sponsor peer into the "black box" of program implementation. While the concern in cell 7 was with the degree to which planned resources were actually delivered, the concern in cell 8 is with the degree to which the planned treatment, or instruction, was delivered to the target population, or the extent to which the materials were used as planned by the target population.

Negative results in cell 10 may mean that the treatment or product was ineffective or that it was not delivered as intended. If the latter is true, then without summative process evaluation the program may be rejected when it may really have been effective. This is analogous to making a Type-I statistical error.

Treatment implementation can be examined through an analysis of records kept over the course of the program such as sign-in sheets, library loan records, case assignment sheets, and teacher activity logs (Morris and Fitz-Gibbon, 1978). Another technique is direct observation with a checklist or observation schedule to record the delivery of key features of the treatment. Interviews and questionnaires can also be profitably used. Such techniques ask participants to report their perceptions of implementation.[5] However, reports of behavior are not as compelling as direct observation of the behavior itself.

Cell 9: Summative Secondary Product Evaluation

One key aspect of any summative evaluation is a review of the product itself independent of its direct effect on recipients. Here the evaluator collects data to answer such questions as how do the content and objectives of the program compare to competitive programs? How do members of the staff, recipients, and other concerned publics feel about the program or product? Expert judgments, survey and questionnaire techniques, and direct observation are the most relevant data-collection techniques to answer such questions.

Cell 10: Summative Primary Product Evaluation

For many the ultimate evaluation questions include the following. How have the recipients been changed as a result of the program? How do any changes compare with those attributable to important competing programs? According to Scriven (1974), "All that should be concerning us, surely [is] determining exactly what effects this product had (or most likely had), and evaluating those, whether or not they were intended" (p. 35).

The most obvious and most widely used means of data collection to answer these questions, in the educational context at least, has been that old standby, the paper-and-pencil test. All too often, however, evaluators disregard the issue of the construct validity of such indirect measures. Fifty years ago Tyler pointed out the need to validate indirect measures before they are used, against measures of direct performance (for example, a paper-and-pencil test on the use of a microscope against having the student actually use a microscope to answer certain questions). He went on to point out the necessity of using direct performance indicators whenever indirect measures did not correlate with the direct. Sampling test items across samples of recipients allows an evaluator to gather much more information about programs without overburdening participants.

Simulations are an intermediate step between direct performance appraisal and indirect paper-and-pencil measures. Computer technology makes such simulations much more feasible than previously. Unobstrusive measures of change such as examination of records is another direct and nonreactive technique that can be employed to measure the effect of a program or product on recipients. Qualitative assessment of outcomes through observation and case study techniques should also be considered in assessing the impact of a program on recipients.

Table 6-1 and CME Evaluations

Reviewing the material on CME evaluations prior to the Conference, it seemed to me that the primary emphasis on such evaluations has been on cell 10. However, in evaluating cell 10, it appears that two important outcomes have been overlooked: (1) the doctor's self-confidence in coping with the constantly changing elements in contemporary medicine; (2) the public perception that doctors are "keeping up" which in the long run may be as important an outcome of CME as any increase in physician knowledge or change in practice. Cell 9 seems to be viewed with downright suspicion, and the other cells, particularly along the formative row, have been virtually ignored. The lack of results attributed to CME in some evaluations may be due to program flaws that could have been corrected during the developmental cycle had they been detected. Negative results may be due to factors related to resource allocation (cell 7) or to a failure to properly implement the treatment (cell 8).

Part III: Data Collection and the Standards

There are 16 Standards (see table 6-2) which the Joint Committee for Educational Evaluation (1981) felt were related to collecting information. In this section I shall *briefly* discuss these 16 Standards in terms of data collection with first, an important caveat. The applicability of any one of these Standards to data collection depends on the context of the evaluation. The size, importance, and budget of the evaluation, as well as the degree of cooperation by different audiences, all have a bearing on the extent to which these 16 Standards individually or collectively might apply to data collection in any given evaluation.

Table 6-2. Relevant Standards for Collecting Information

Utility Standards

- A2 Evaluator Credibility
- A3 Information Scope and Selection

Feasibility Standards

- A4 Valuational Interpretation
- B1 Practical Procedures

Propriety Standards

- B2 Political Viability
- C1 Formal Obligation
- C5 Rights of Human Subjects
- C6 Human Interactions

Accuracy Standards

- C7 Balanced Reporting
- D1 Object Identification
- D2 Context Analysis
- D3 Described Purposes and Procedures
- D4 Defensible Information Sources
- D5 Valid Measurement
- D6 Reliable Measurement
- D7 Systematic Data Control

Utility Standards and Data Collection

Three of the Utility Standards, all of which are intended to ensure that an evaluation serves the practical information needs of given audiences, have direct applicability to data collection. The first, *Evaluator Credibility,* speaks to whether or not the evaluator has the training and technical competence to collect the data needed to answer the questions of concern. This Standard again raises the issue of the evaluator's biases and world view discussed in Part I. For large evaluations, no single person may have all the necessary technical skills to insure evaluator credibility. An evaluation team may be the only way to meet this standard.

The second Utility Standard, *Information Scope and Selection,* requires that the data collected address pertinent questions and be responsive to the needs and interests of specified audiences. The evaluator needs to identify the information needs of important audiences and then work with the client and representatives of the various audiences to put in priority order these often quite diverse information needs. In deciding on priority of information needs, Cronbach (1982) argues that the evaluator needs to consider each information request in terms of "leverage," that is, how much influence is each of the conceivable answers to this research question expected to have? (p. 226).

One aspect of leverage is political: does an important bloc want an answer? Will the answer sway an important uncommitted group? A second aspect of leverage is scope: high priority goes to information needs that address large issues rather than details. A third aspect of leverage is that the information is value-laden for at least some members of the policy-shaping groups. Finally, Cronbach (1982) argues that the evaluator, by his/her choice of data to be collected, "should open the door to neglected values . . . to bring in the questions and interests of groups that are comparatively powerless, notably the disadvantaged" (p. 229).

The last Utility Standard of interest in data collection is that of *Valuation Interpretation.* The perspectives, procedures, and rationale used to interpret the findings should be carefully described so that the bases for value judgments are clear. Among other things, this Standard speaks to the value orientation of the evaluator, as discussed in Part I. It also requires that consideration be given to the use of alternative data-collection techniques to answer the same question. Different techniques used to answer a single question can result in quite different information and value meanings, thereby substantially altering the inferences made about the program, project or product.

Feasibility Standards and Data Collection

Feasibility Standards require that an evaluator be realistic, prudent, diplomatic and frugal in his/her work (Joint Committee, 1981). Two Standards, *Political Procedures* and *Political Viability*, speak, in part, to the task of data collection. The first reminds the evaluator that data-collection techniques which they use be practical and keep disruption to a minimum. Data-collection techniques should be chosen so that they can be implemented within the constraints of time, budget, and participant availability and cooperation. Before techniques are finalized they should be reviewed by participants, clients, and other concerned publics as to their practicality and political viability.

The second Feasibility Standard requires that data collection be planned and conducted anticipating the different political and value positions held by various concerned audiences. In this way cooperation can be obtained, and possible attempts to curtail the evaluation or misapply results, forestalled. Additionally, this Standard reminds evaluators to negotiate a contract which makes explicit the evaluator's right of access to the required data. The contract should also spell out, as far as possible, the obligations of the client and other concerned parties, to cooperate in providing the necessary data identified as part of the Information Scope and Selection.

Propriety Standards and Data Collection

Four of the Propriety Standards are directly applicable to the task of data collection (i.e., C1, C5, C6, C7). As a group, these four Standards require the evaluator to implement data-collection techniques which are legal and ethical, and which respect the welfare and rights of those involved in the evaluation.

The first of these, *Formal Obligations,* requires that the parties to an evaluation agree in writing to what is to be done, how, by whom, and when. More specifically, the written agreement should include (1) the data-collection plan along with a description of the data, sources of data, sample size and selection, instrumentation, and other techniques used to gather data; (2) the time schedule for collection of the data; and (3) the methods for assuring quality control during data collection.

The second Propriety Standard, *Rights of Human Subjects,* requires that data collection be designed so that the rights and welfare of those affected are respected and protected. Specifically, in collecting data the evaluator must (1) obtain appropriate written permission from the subjects (or their parents or legal guardians) or relevant administrators for access to individual records; (2) obtain informed consent when administering certain instruments or using certain techniques; (3) set up procedures to protect, when necessary, the anonymity of those who supply data; (4) set in place safeguards against other parties using the information collected for purposes different from those agreed to by the persons from whom the data were collected; (5) communicate unambiguously how the information persons provide will be used, and the extent to which it will be kept confidential; and (6) avoid data-collection methods that have a potential for violating the rights of those affected.

The third Propriety Standard, *Human Interaction,* requires that evaluators respect the dignity and worth of individuals when collecting data. Here the evaluator should consider *not* collecting information which might embarrass participants if it is not absolutely essential, or when it is essential, collecting it in ways which would protect the identity of those giving the information.

The final Propriety Standard that impinges directly on data collection is *Balanced Reporting.* Specifically, when relevant data are inaccessible because of cost or other constraints, such omissions need to be reported; a discussion of their effect on the overall judgment of the program, if they were either strongly positive or negative, should be developed and presented in the final report.

Accuracy Standards and Data Collection

The first seven Accuracy Standards are directly applicable to the job of data collection. In general, all address the need to ensure that the judgment of the merit or worth of the program, or project, will be based on technically adequate information. As a group, these Standards are a constant reminder of the principle that judgments about a program based on invalid, unreliable data are themselves not valid. The hackneyed acronym G.I.G.O. (gargage in; garbage out) sums up this scene.

The first Accuracy Standard, *Object Identification,* requires that before data are collected the object of the evaluation be clearly identified and defined. This Standard requires that the evaluator check not just with the client but with other concerned audiences on their perceptions of what it is that is being evaluated before designing data-collection techniques. Often, different publics will see the program in quite different ways, and consequently have quite different information needs. These different perceptions themselves are interesting and valuable data, and should be presented in the report. Data on these perceptions can be obtained from interviews, minutes, proposals, public relation reports, press clippings, etc. As the evaluation unfolds, the evaluator also needs to be attentive to any changes in the way concerned publics view the program or project. Perceptions change for many reasons, one of which may be the intrusion of the evaluators and their data-collection techniques.

The second Accuracy Standard, *Context Analysis,* relates to cells 1 and 6, discussed earlier. It requires that the social, political, and economic context of the program, or project, should be identified not only as sources of data in themselves but also in order to anticipate any influence that they may have on either the collection or interpretation of data.

The third Accuracy Standard, *Described Purposes and Procedures,* and the fourth, *Defensible Information Sources,* can be considered jointly. These Standards require that the evaluator describe in the report the details of the data-collection techniques (i.e., sources, sample, instrumentation, schedule, etc.) so they can be identified and assessed. Sample attrition, any deviation from planned data-collection procedures, and the reasons for any such changes should be documented. Copies of all instruments and procedures should be included in an appendix. The purposes of both Standards are to ensure adequate documentation of how data were collected. Such documentation permits reviews and evaluations of what was done and makes possible secondary analysis of the data by others. In short, these Standards require an audit trail of the data-collection phase of the evaluation.

The fifth Accuracy Standard, *Valid Measurement,* goes to the heart of data collection and data interpretation. The Standard requires that evaluators describe (1) the content and constructs measured; (2) validity information, both quantitative and qualitative, on instruments or procedures purporting to measure particular content and constructs; and (3) how the instruments or procedures were administered, scored or coded, and interpreted.

Standard D5 reminds the evaluator that validity is specific; that validity inheres not in the instrument itself but in the interpretation made from using the instrument with a particular population to answer a particular question. Standard D5 also points to the need for multiple imperfect measures of multiple outcomes rather than the overreliance on a single data-collection technique. No program or project — or individual for that matter — can or should be characterized or assessed by reference to a single measure. Very often the validity of using paper-and-pencil measures in an evaluation is taken for granted or never discussed.[6] Yet the validity of the inferences one makes about the merit or worth of a program are based, in important part, on the validity of the inferences made from the instruments used to collect the data in the first place.[7] Because of this it is important that an evaluator document the reasons for choosing an extant instrument and provide validity data on any instrument built especially for the program, so that the appropriateness of the instrument and the validity of the inferences can themselves be evaluated.

The sixth Accuracy Standard, *Reliable Measurement,* requires that information-gathering instruments and procedures — whether quantitative or qualitative — be chosen or developed in ways that will assure that the information obtained is reliable or consistent. There is a variety of procedures for estimating reliability. Therefore, the procedures chosen depend on the way in which the data will be aggregated and used. In some cases, the consistency and/or stability of individual scores are at issue. In other cases, the consistency of individual decisions made on the basis of a cut score is at issue. In still other cases, the reliability of the average score of a group is of primary concern, and traditional methods of estimating reliability can be misleading. The chosen reliability index (or indices) should be justified in terms of the intended use to which instrument is put.

The final Accuracy Standard, *Systematic Data Control,* reminds the evaluator to check continually for errors in collecting, scoring, coding, recording, collating, key-punching, and analyzing data. Data can be compromised at any number of points in an evaluation. This Standard reminds us of one of Murphy's Laws that "anything that can go wrong probably will" (Joint Committee, 1981, p. 124). The Standard in effect requires of the evaluator a systematic program of training those collecting or processing the data, and systematic controls and accuracy checks throughout the entire process.

Data Standards and CME Evaluation

How do the Standards relate to data collection for CME evaluations? The Standards provide guidelines that clients commissioning an evaluation of a CME project can use to evaluate the evaluator and the work of the evaluator at every stage in the process. For the evaluator of a CME project, the Standards provide a set of guidelines of good practice that go way beyond data collection. For both clients and evaluator, the Standards highlight the need to involve all concerned publics in the task of defining the evaluation questions, and in choosing the data-collection techniques to answer these questions.

Conclusion

This chapter has discussed data collection from three perspectives. First from a philosophical or value perspective, the type of data collected and the techniques used to collect them are a function of the evaluator's frame of reference: his/her philosophy of evaluation. We argued that evaluations too often have wrongly tried to apply the technique of the natural sciences to the evaluation of social program and that there is a need, for CME evaluations, to be open to other modes of inquiry.

Second, how the role of the evaluator affects data collection was discussed. The data needs and techniques used vary with the nature of the evaluation — whether it is formative or summative or context-, input-, process-, or product-oriented. Finally we considered briefly each of the 16 Standards applicable to data collection.

I would like to close with the words of Richard LaPierre who, writing in 1928, observed, "The study of human behavior is time-consuming, intellectually fatiguing, and depends for its success upon the ability of the investigator. . . . Quantitative measures are quantitatively accurate; qualitative evaluations are always subject to the errors of human judgment. Yet it would seem far more worthwhile to make a shrewd guess regarding that which is essential than to accurately measure that which is likely to prove quite irrelevant" (p. 237). A shrewd guess would be that today's discerning project directors, particularly in CME, would bypass Friday, Holmes, and Gradgrind of DATAFAX, INC., in favor of the newly formed and yet-to-be-named firm of Columbo, Father Brown, and Miss Marple.

Notes

1. When Jack Webb died recently, his obituaries included comments from police officials regarding his portrayal of Joe Friday. Some appreciated Friday's emphasis on the facts because it projected for them an image of concern for hard evidence. At the same time other police officials were concerned with that because the unsmiling Friday's emphasis on facts projected an image of the policeman as unconcerned with the personal situation of individuals caught up in a police situation.

2. Whatever is received is received after the manner of the receiver.

3. While there are important ideological differences among evaluators holding different conceptualizations of evaluation, it should be noted that among those who purport to hold the same conceptualization of evaluation there are also important differences in the methods used to collect data and in the data actually collected.

4. For a full treatment of needs assessment in the areas of health and human services see *Evaluation and Program Planning,* (1981). Special Needs Assessment Issue, 4(1).

5. See Morris, L.L. and FitzGibbon, C.T. (1978). *How to measure program implementation.* Beverly Hills: Sage Publications. This contains a full description of the data techniques for program implementation.

6. For a discussion of the validity of commercially available standardized texts used in program evaluations, see chapters 5 and 6 in Madaus, G.F., Airasian, P.W., and Kellaghan, T. (1980). *School effectiveness: A reassessment of the evidence.* New York: McGraw-Hill Book Company. Also the APA, AERA, and NCME Committee to Develop Joint Technical Stan-

dards for Educational and Psychological Testing is in the process of developing Technical Standards for the use of tests in program evaluation. When these Standards are eventually published they will complement and supplement the Accuracy Standards of the Joint Committee on Standards for Educational Evaluation.

7. It is difficult to separate the use of particular instruments from issues of design and statistical analysis; ultimately the validity of inferences made about a program depends on all these factors.

References

Cronbach, L.J. (1982). *Designing evaluations of education and social programs.* San Francisco: Jossey-Bass.

Deutscher, I. (1976). "Words and deeds: Social science and social policy." In W.B. Sanders (ed.), *The sociologist as detective. An introduction to research methods.* New York: Praeger.

Dickens, C. (1981). *Hard Times.* New York: Bantam Books. (Original work published in 1854.)

Doyle, A.C. (1981). "A scandal in Bohemia." In J. Symons (ed.), *The complete adventures of Sherlock Holmes.* London: Secker and Warburg.

Fink, A. and Kosecoff, J. (1983). "How to evaluate cost effectiveness." *How to evaluate education programs,* 65, 1–7.

Joint Committee on Standards for Educational Evaluation. (1981). Standards for evaluation of educational programs, projects, and materials. New York: McGraw-Hill.

LaPierre, R.T. (1928). "Race prejudice: France and England." *Social Forces,* 7, 102–111.

Levin, H.M. (1974). "Cost effectiveness analysis in evaluation research." *Evaluation Consortium,* Stanford: Stanford University Press.

Lloyd, A.L. (1967). *Folk song in England.* Great Britain: Lawrence and Wishart.

Lloyd, J.S. and Abrahamson, S. (1979). "Effectiveness of continuing medical education: A review of the evidence." *Evaluation and the Health Professions,* 2(3), 251–280.

Madaus, G.F. and McDonagh, J.T. (1982). "As I roved out: Folksong collecting as a metaphor for evaluation." In N.L. Smith (ed.), *Communication strategies in evaluation.* Beverly Hills: Sage Publications.

Medawar, P. (1982). *Pluto's Republic.* New York: Oxford University Press.

Morris, L.L. and Fitz-Gibbon, C.T. (1978). *How to measure program implementation.* Beverly Hills: Sage Publications.

Perry, W.G., Jr. (1967). "Examsmanship and the liberal arts: A study in educational epistemology." In M.C. Beardsley (ed.), *Modes of argument.* Indianapolis: Bobbs-Merrill Educational Publishing.

Scriven, M. (1973). "The methodology of education." In B.R. Worthen and J.R. Sanders (eds.), *Educational evaluation: Theory and practice.* Belmont, California: Charles A. Jones.

Scriven, M. (1974). "Pros and cons about goal-free evaluation." In W.J. Popham (ed.), *Evaluation in education.* Berkeley: McCutchan Publishing.

Snow, C.P. (1962). *The two cultures: And a second look.* Glasgow: Blackie and Son, Ltd.

Sibley, J.C., Sackett, D.L., Neufeld, V., Gerrard, B., Rudnick, K.V., and Fraser, W. (1982). "A randomized trial of continuing medical education." *New England Journal of Medicine,* 306(9), 511–515.

Spector, R.D. (1981). Introduction to *Hard times.* New York: Bantam Books.

Stufflebeam, D. (1973). "An introduction to the PDK book: Educational evaluation and decision making." In B.R. Worthen and J.R. Sanders (eds.), *Educational evaluation: Theory and practice.* Belmont, California: Charles A. Jones.

Stufflebeam, D. (1983). "The CIPP model for program evaluation." In G.F. Madaus, M. Scriven, and D. Stufflebeam (eds.), *Evaluation models.* Hingham, Massachusetts: Kluwer-Nijhoff Publishing.

Thomas, L. (1979). *The Medusa and the snail: More notes of a biology watcher.* New York: Bantam Books.

7 DATA-COLLECTION TECHNIQUES IN EVALUATION

Julie G. Nyquist

Understanding of any complex process such as evaluation is facilitated by looking at one piece of the total process at a time. Data collection, as one phase of evaluation, is the focus of this chapter. It must, however, be emphasized that it is really not possible to discuss any one phase in isolation. All decisions within the evaluation process are interrelated and dependent on both earlier and subsequent decisions. So while the discussion here focuses on data collection, we need to retain our perspective of it as only one aspect of evaluation, interrelated with others.

This chapter is divided into three sections. The first is a discussion of a variety of issues related to data collection, including (1) an analysis of the impact of the evaluator's frame of reference, (2) the relationship of formative and summative evaluation to data collection, and (3) the multiple approaches to deciding what kinds of data should be collected. The second section examines actual data-collection techniques which could be used in evaluation of continuing education in the health professions. The final section provides critical commentary related to the Standards and data collection.

Issues Related to Data Collection

Evaluator's Frame of Reference

Evaluation is a subject as well as an objective process, involving judgment in all phases of planning and implementation. It is therefore logical that an evaluator's frame of reference will have an impact — throughout the evaluation process — on the determination of design, data-collection methods, analysis, and reporting. Madaus, in his chapter, discussed one view of frame of reference, contrasting two polar positions: (1) the traditional/positivistic/quantitative approach to evaluation and (2) the recently emerging phenomenological/qualitative approach. He noted that the first group emphasizes application of the "scientific method" and collection of quantifiable data. In contrast, the second group emphasizes the concept that the whole is greater than the sum of the parts, and stresses that evaluation should help the client and key publics to better understand a program, therefore collecting a variety of quantifiable and nonquantifiable data. Madaus recommends that a mix of approaches should result in a more useful and more valid evaluation, but notes that this would add to the cost of any evaluation.

At the Conference in discussion of these two approaches, participant comments indicated a belief that the phenomenological/qualitative approach presented more potential problems than the traditional approach. Three basic concerns were expressed. First, when the purpose of the evaluation is basically a research purpose (i.e., to add to the cumulative knowledge about the effectiveness of particular continuing-education approaches), the participants were concerned with the political issue of credibility. This refers to the credibility of the data and results, in the eyes of critical audiences (i.e., journal editors, funding agencies, and other researchers). The second concern was also politically based. The feeling of some participants was that frequently the orientation and biases of those commissioning evaluation of continuing education in the health professions (CE) preclude the possibility of the evaluator's even considering the use of a phenomenological approach. The approach and its benefits may need to be promoted before it can be suggested for use in an evaluation study in CE. The final concern was that qualitative data alone would often not provide a sufficient basis for making objective decisions about a program. Most of the participants would probably agree with Madaus that a mix of approaches is best; but when financial constraints are severe, a clear objectives-based approach would generally be selected.

Regardless of the arguments for or against the specific perspectives discussed, one thing seems very clear: an evaluator, in an applied area like evaluation of continuing education in the health professions, cannot afford the luxury of having a rigid or polar frame of reference. This caveat extends beyond the dimension of quantitative-versus-qualitative to any other dimension (e.g., personal, political, educational) which might affect one's total frame of reference and result in rigidity of application of any specific approach to evaluation. The evaluator must be a generalist, aware of varied approaches and willing to modify them in order to collect useful data relevant to the particular purpose of each separate evaluation effort. Frame of reference is only one factor affecting the design of evaluation efforts. It is the design itself which should dictate what types of data will be collected and how.

Formative and Summative Evaluation

The distinction between formative and summative evaluation is frequently stressed in the literature of educational evaluation. However, most of the programs to be evaluated extend over a set period of time and have a stable and relatively homogeneous group of participants. These conditions often do not exist in continuing education in the health professions; programs vary from one-hour, one-shot lectures to extended individualized learning programs. A discussion of formative evaluation in CE contexts makes sense only when programs are of sufficient length and continuity to make formative changes possible. The Conference participants particularly questioned the usefulness of the formative/summative distinction for evaluation within traditional information-dissemination, lecture-based courses.

Again, it must be stressed that it is the purpose of a program evaluation and the specific questions to be answered by it that determine the data-collection plan, i.e., what data, how collected, when, and from whom. The formative/summative distinction is one of several that can help guide these decisions as well as other design, analysis, and interpretation decisions.

Determining What Kinds of Data to Collect

There are many different ways to view data. Each method provides a slightly different perspective and set of insights which may be useful in the decision-making phase of an evaluation process. Four of these possible ways to decide what kinds of data to collect are discussed briefly below.

1. Learning Outcomes. Data collection can be based upon the learning outcomes of interest. In CE there are four basic types of learning outcomes discussed in the literature: learner satisfaction; change in knowledge, attitudes, or skills of learners; change in the practice behaviors of learners; and change in the health status of patients. All four outcomes are assumed to relate more or less directly to the ultimate goal of CE which is to improve both the quality of health care and the health status of patients. Clearly the first two classes of outcome relate to intermediate objectives which, in turn, must be assumed to relate to changes in practice and/or changes in health status. However, reliable assessment is increasingly difficult and costly to obtain as we move from learner satisfaction toward changes in patient health. It is also difficult to eliminate alternative explanations (i.e., other than CE) for any changes demonstrated.

In preparing this chapter I conducted a thorough survey of 48 reports of CE evaluation studies published in the years 1973–1983. This survey incorporated all of the post-1972 studies discussed in the classic Lloyd and Abrahamson review (1979), all eight of the studies reviewed by Stein (1981), several studies from the Bertram and Brooks-Bertram review (1977), plus studies from evaluation of CE in other health professions. Typical forms of data collection vary according to learning outcome. For learner satisfaction the typical measure is a postcourse questionnaire (Miller et al., 1978; Holzemer et al., 1980; Woog and Hyman, 1980; Petersen, 1982). To assess changes in knowledge, attitudes, or skills, the typical measures are (1) for knowledge, an objective examination (Hazlett et al., 1973; Rubenstein, 1973; Neu and Howrey, 1975; Chambers et al., 1976; Miller et al., 1978; Kattwinkel et al., 1979; Sula et al., 1979; Wang et al., 1979; Harlan et al., 1980; Holzemer et al., 1980; Woog and Hyman, 1980; Dickinson et al., 1981; Richardson, 1981; Petersen, 1982); (2) for attitudes, some form of attitude inventory (Brennan et al., 1974; Durlack and Burchard, 1977; Kattwinkel et al., 1979; Woog and Hyman, 1980; Richardson, 1981); and (3) for skills, an observational assessment instrument (Holzemer et al., 1980). For changes in practice behaviors, the typical instrument is a focused pre- and posteducation chart audit (Ashbaugh and McKean, 1976; Bird, 1976; Innui et al., 1976; McDonald, 1976; Nelson, 1976; Payne et al., 1976; DeVitt, 1973; Reed et al., 1973; Rubenstein, 1973; Cayten et al., 1974; DeBombal et al., 1974; DeVitt and Ironside, 1975; Grimm et al., 1975; Laxdall et al., 1978; Talley, 1978; Kattwinkel et al., 1979; Harlan et al., 1980; Avorn and Soumerai, 1983; Gullion et al., 1983; Rosser, 1983), but other techniques are used as well. Examples of techniques include review of hospital pharmacy or laboratory records (Eisenberg et al., 1977; West et al., 1977); review of charges or claim records (Schroeder et al., 1973; Buck and White, 1974; Williamson et al., 1975; Brook and Williams, 1976), survey of patients or supervisors to assess change (Condon 1974; Woog and Hyman, 1980; Little et al., 1983), use of log diaries to record behavior and assess change (Jewell and Schneiderman, 1978), direct observation of behavior using a structured recording instrument (Chambers, 1976; Holzemer et al., 1980), and survey of participants to obtain self-reports of change, either by questionnaire (Caplan, 1973; Inui et al., 1976; Jewell and Schneiderman, 1978; Miller et al., 1978; Wang et al., 1979; Petersen, 1982; Little et al., 1983); or interview (Miller et al., 1978; Richardson, 1981). To determine changes in patient health status, most techniques involve use of patient records to assess specific aspects of health (Williamson et al., 1975; Inui et al., 1976; Dickinson et al., 1981; Gullion et al., 1983), although questionnaires or content examinations can be given to patients to assess some types of changes (Inui et al., 1976).

The Conference participants expressed a sense of frustration that too often the only evaluation possible, given typical time and monetary constraints, is assessment of learner satisfaction. To counter this difficult problem some participants recommended that more research be done in units like the USC Development and Demonstration Center where it is possible to include data collection related to all four types of learning outcomes and investigate the linkages among them.

2. Madaus's Model.   Another method of determining what data to collect is to use a formal educational evaluation model. Various models have been developed and are in frequent use (Worthen and Sanders, 1973). Madaus, in his chapter, has presented a comprehensive model which combines features of Stufflebeam's and Scriven's models. The result is a model with ten cells, five formative and five summative. Each cell is described in detail by Madaus, along with the types of data-collection methods appropriate within each cell; the model need not be repeated here.

In discussion of the Madaus model, Conference participants generally felt that it provided a useful way of thinking about the varied aspects of program development and implementation which could be evaluated; that is, it provided a new perspective for some. However, many felt that to use this model in real CE evaluation situations would generally be unrealistic, especially in low-budget and/or one-shot programs. Participants particularly questioned their ability to gather data in cells 3 (formative process evaluation), 4 (formative secondary product evaluation), 5 (formative primary product evaluation), and 6 (summative context evaluation) during typical one-shot, lecture-based CE programs.

In his general commentary on CME evaluation and his model, Madaus observed that the primary emphasis in CME evaluation has been on cell 10 (summative primary product evaluation). Although this is true, data are frequently collected in other cells as well. In my survey of 48 reports of CE evaluation studies, 18 were reports of individualized CE programs. In the vast majority of these cases, a needs assessment was an integral part of the program (cell 1), and in cases where written materials were part of the treatment, an expert analysis prior to use was also reported. Also, although there is undoubtedly truth in Madaus's comment that "Cell nine (summative secondary product evaluation) seemed to be viewed with downright suspicion," cell-9 data are often collected. In fact it is possible that Madaus was reacting to the frustration expressed by many CE evaluators that the *only* data they have the time and money to collect are participant opinions about the program (cell 9) separate from the program's effects on the participants. This reflects not so much a suspicion of program data as a desire to go beyond program-related data to collect relevant cell-10 data so that effects can also be assessed.

3. Cognitive, Affective, and Psychomotor Domains.   Throughout educational literature, particularly that dealing with educational objectives, there are references to educational taxonomies, especially that developed by Bloom (1956). Bloom's taxonomy divided educational objectives into three domains: cognitive, affective, and psychomotor. Taxonomies are useful in making decisions about the types of data to collect when the program goals relate directly to learner characteristics in the cognitive, affective, or psychomotor domains. For example, if one goal of a CE program is to "transmit" information, an assessment instrument (e.g., an objective test) will generally be developed for use. A taxonomy can be used to help guide decisions about what levels to assess: knowledge, comprehension, application, analysis, synthesis, or evaluation. Use of a taxonomy in instances like this can be helpful. The taxonomy can also be used to assess whether CE studies address application issues or merely knowledge and comprehension of information. However, in CE the truly desired focus is most often on changing the behaviors of health professionals. Although most behaviors have cognitive, affective, and psychomotor components, it is generally the behavior, and not the components, that is of interest. In fact, it is often difficult to define the separate components. So while use of Bloom's taxonomy, or any other taxonomy, could add depth to evaluation studies which focus specifically on changes in knowledge, attitudes, or skills, this distinction has less potential use for assessment of behavior changes.

4. Products versus Behaviors.   Another type of distinction that can be used when deciding what kinds of data to collect is the product-versus-behaviors distinction. As has been stated, change in behavior is most frequently the primary focus of CE. However, there are occasions — especially in dental CE — when a particular product could be the focus of assessment. Also, charts and records are frequently used as data sources and both could be considered products.

Other Issues

1. Direct versus Indirect Assessment. One data-collection issue that faces evaluators in CE is whether to use direct or indirect assessment of important dependent variables. Typically, learner satisfaction and change in learner knowledge or attitudes are assessed as directly as possible using paper-and-pencil instruments. However, learner behaviors of health-care providers in their natural settings are assessed more frequently through indirect measures. In my review of recent CE evaluation studies, 38 assessed changes in behavior. Of these, only 2 reported using direct observation of health professionals while 1 other directly assessed drug-prescribing patterns using subscription slips. Contrarily, there were 38 instances of use of indirect measures including chart audit (20 studies), review of other records (5 studies), self-report of changes using questionnaires (8 studies), self-report of changes using interviews (2 studies), and reports of changes by peers, patients, or supervisors (3 studies).

The major advantage of direct assessment is that it allows for very specific and in-depth assessment of specified performances. The disadvantages, particularly for direct observation, include obtrusiveness, high cost and time requirements, and the difficulty in assessing across time and across cases. Because these disadvantages are also relative advantages of indirect measures, particularly chart or record audit, the current trend of using these measures appears sound.

2. Natural versus Controlled Stimulus Situations. Another data-collection decision facing evaluators of CE is whether data should be collected in naturally occurring settings or in controlled-stimulus (or simulated) situations. There are three basic types of controlled-stimulus situations: (1) live, using simulated or programmed patients and direct observation; (2) paper-and-pencil or computer simulations of clinical problems; and (3) models used to assess physical-examination, technical, or production skills. In training situations within medical and health-professions education, controlled-stimulus situations have been used to great advantage in assessment of varied clinical skills. However, within evaluation of CE, assessment has been done almost exclusively within naturally occurring situations.

None of the 48 studies that I reviewed reported using simulation techniques; however, several earlier studies used patient management problems (Manning et al., 1968; McClellan and Cox, 1968), a simulated certification examination (Naftulin and Ware, 1971) to assess clinical problem-solving, and an interview to assess interpersonal skills (Bacal, 1971).

This is one area, especially in an era of advanced computer applications, where evaluation of CE might be enhanced by increased consideration of the possibilities for use of controlled-stimulus situations, especially in funded evaluation research of continuing education.

3. Data Collection and Needs Assessment. Several recent discussions of continuing medical education have emphasized the importance of needs assessment as part of the processes of planning and evaluating CE (Stein, 1981; Laxdall, 1982). Data collection is an essential part of the needs-assessment phase of any major CE program or program evaluation.

There are two main types of learning needs. Perceived needs represent the perspective of the learners, while actual or "true" needs are more objectively determined by independent assessment using factually recorded data. Data to determine perceived needs are usually gathered with the use of some type of self-report questionnaire. Data related to actual or "true" needs are usually gathered from reviews of charts or laboratory, pharmacy, or hospital records.

The importance of data collection at the needs-assessment phase was emphasized by Stein (1981) in his analysis of eight CME studies, all using needs assessment of some form and all showing positive changes in physician performance (Caplan, 1973; Buck and White, 1974; Inui et al., 1976; Laxdall et al., 1978; Mahan et al., 1978; Talley, 1978; Kattwinkel et al., 1979; Wang et al., 1979).

Techniques of Data Collection

A wide variety of data-collection techniques have been used in evaluation of continuing-education programs. A brief discussion of several techniques is provided here. Each discussion will include examples of the variables assessed by the technique along with a description of the advantages and disadvantages or cautions for each usage.

Content Examinations

Content examinations are used frequently in CE to assess gains in knowledge (Jones and Taxay, 1963; Gauvain et al., 1965; Cameron, 1966; Menzel et al., 1966; Meyer, 1967; Edson et al., 1969; Tucker and Reinhardt, 1969; Caplan, 1971; Naftulin and Ware, 1971; Donnelly et al., 1972; Driver et al., 1972; Hazlett et al., 1973; Rubenstein, 1973; Neu and Howrey, 1975; Chambers et al., 1976; Miller et al., 1978; Kattwinkel et al., 1979; Sula et al., 1979; Wang et al., 1979; Harlan et al., 1980; Holzemer et al., 1980; Woog and Hyman, 1980; Dickinson et al., 1981; Richardson, 1981; Petersen, 1982), and well-written, appropriately used objective tests can provide a good measure of knowledge for any carefully defined content area. Objective tests can have the advantages of content validity, convenience of administration and scoring, and relatively high reliability. However, to have these advantages, examinations must be carefully prepared and based upon clear content objectives. Further, when examinations are used both precourse and postcourse, there are several cautions: (1) the possibility exists that some participants may fake poor performance on a pretest in order to maximize apparent gain in knowledge; (2) there may be interactions between the pretest and the CE experience, making it very difficult to be certain that any measured gains in knowledge can be attributed to the experience alone. Finally, when examinations are used to collect data in evaluation of CE, the report of results should include information about how the test was selected or constructed (e.g., if it was compared to objectives and reviewed by experts), as well as data about the level and type of reliability statistics calculated for each administration.

Attitude Inventories

Attitude inventories of varying types, generally designed by the program evaluators, are used to assess attitude change in some CE evaluation studies (Forman et al., 1964; Tucker and Reinhardt, 1969; Mock et al., 1970; Donnelly et al., 1972; Brennan et al., 1977; Durlack and Burchard, 1977; Kattwinkel et al., 1979; Woog and Hyman, 1980; Richardson, 1981). Although attitude inventories have the advantage of being relatively easy and inexpensive to develop, administer, and score, they have the severe disadvantages of generally unknown or questionable reliability and validity. Use of inventories also assumes that participants have both the ability and desire to answer the items honestly. Considering the disadvantages of this technique, it is recommended that it be used only in studies using multiple techniques for data collection.

Survey Techniques

The two basic survey techniques used in the evaluation of CE programs are questionnaires and interviews. The questionnaire technique has the advantages of convenience of self-administration, relatively low cost, and ease of scoring. Questionnaires have the disadvantage of inability to question in depth. If mailed to subjects, they also have the disadvantages of risk of low returns, and inability to assure that questions are understood and answered as intended. Interviews have the advantage of the possibility of questioning in depth. Interviews, however, have the disadvantages of relatively high cost and large time commitment needed for administration and scoring.

These survey techniques are used to collect a variety of data in CE evaluation. Questionnaires are the primary means used to assess participant reaction to or satisfaction with CE programs. Although not often reported in the literature (Miller et al., 1978; Holzemer et al., 1980; Woog and Hyman, 1980; Petersen, 1982), this is still the most common assessment instrument used in evaluation of CE programs. This technique is most appropriately used to screen out particularly bad program sessions or for gathering suggestions for future program improvements. Few persons would rely on these data alone as valid indicators of program achievement.

Questionnaires can, however, address other issues such as participant opinions about achievement of course objectives, and *intended* changes in practice behaviors (Caplan, 1973; Inui et al., 1976). In the same vein, questionnaires are used to obtain an indirect measure of behavioral change. The most commonly used measures are participant self-report questionnaires (Garfin, 1969; Boeck et al., 1972; Caplan, 1973; Inui et al., 1976; Jewell and Schneiderman, 1978; Miller et al., 1978; Wang et al., 1979; Petersen, 1982; Little et al., 1983), but are also used occasionally as questionnaires completed by peers (Woog and Hyman, 1980), supervisors (Condon, 1974), or patients (Woog and Hyman, 1980; Little et al., 1983). Self-report questionnaires, whether completed by care-providers, peers, supervisors, or patients, clearly have the potential for providing useful information. They must, however, be carefully prepared, linked to objectives, and written with the understanding that the respondents must *both* have the information asked for *and* be willing to provide it accurately and honestly. Use of questionnaires to gather behavioral data is particularly appropriate when more direct measures (e.g., direct observation, chart review) are not feasible due to cost, time, or other constraints.

Interviews are used much less frequently in evaluation of CE programs. In general, the disadvantages of the higher cost and greater time commitment required have outweighed the advantages. Advantages of interviews include the following: (1) flexibility is increased, allowing questions to be repeated and clarified if they are not at first understood; (2) literacy on the part of the respondent is not required; and (3) respondents are generally amenable to questioning in a sensitive area since the interviewer can put a respondent at ease and can note nonverbal as well as verbal cues. With well-trained interviewers and well-designed recording instruments, the advantages above could be put to good use with some patient populations, to gather data about the behaviors of health-care providers or about patients' current health status. However, none of the studies surveyed reported using interviews in this manner. Only two studies, of those surveyed, reported using interviews, both in an effort to determine from learners if any practice behaviors had changed as a result of CE programs (Dickinson et al., 1981; Richardson, 1981).

Observational Techniques

In the context of evaluation of CE, observational techniques are generally used to assess two things: acquisition of clinical skills (Bacal, 1971; Naftulin and Ware, 1971; Shepherd, 1971; Holzemer et al., 1980), and changes in practitioner behaviors (Chambers, 1976). The most commonly used obervational techniques can be divided into two categories: (1) direct observation of specific skills or behaviors and (2) ratings of habitual performance. Acquisition of clinical skills is appropriately assessed through direct observation, either in natural or controlled settings. The more general category of practitioner behaviors can be assessed by ratings of habitual performance (completed by self, peers, supervisors, or patients), or through direct observation in natural or controlled settings.

In the above section on survey techniques, questionnaires used indirectly to assess changes in practitioner behaviors were mentioned. Questionnaires of this type can also be classified as indirect observational instruments when they include ratings of habitual performance, to be completed by the practitioner, supervisor, peer, or patient. Ratings of this type have the advantage of providing a relatively inexpensive means of obtaining information about the quality of performance changes that might be related to CE program involvement.

There are, however, drawbacks to use of this type of instrument. The primary drawback relates to rater errors, including constant errors like generosity error, where the rater tends to rate everyone as better than average, and the problem of halo effect, where a rater who is positively (or negatively) impressed with one aspect of the practitioner lets this impression affect ratings of all other aspects. Other possible difficulties include ambiguity of items and the likelihood that some raters will not have all of the information requested. All of these problems are exacerbated if it is not possible to train the raters and/or if the raters have had limited contact with the practitioner.

A good data-collection plan is essential if ratings of habitual performance are to provide valid information. To maximize the usefulness of information obtained, the plan should include (1) specifications for selection of raters that consider amount of previous contact with the practitioner and types of information needed from the raters, and (2) provision for use of multiple raters, to maximize reliability of information and minimize the effect of rating errors and biases.

Direct observation is a particularly useful source of data regarding the processes of health care. Accompanied by use of a structured assessment instrument, it is the most highly recommended technique for assessment of clinical skills, including interviewing, conduct of physical examinations, and performance of technical skills. Observation is a very powerful tool for teaching as well as evaluation. This is particularly true when performances are recorded on videotape, which allows (1) both the learner and instructor the opportunity to review the performance and (2) the evaluator or researcher the opportunity to check the reliability of ratings and provide rater training. In fact, observation is essential to the processes of teaching and learning clinical skills.

Direct observation does, however, have several disadvantages as a technique for evaluation of CE. First, it requires a considerable amount of professional time, and optimally would require two or more observers. It also requires training of the observers and careful preparation and testing of the recording or rating instrument. This is necessary in order to assure agreement on scoring criteria and encourage high interrater reliability. There is also a caution associated with the use of direct observation: being observed can affect practitioner performance. Health-care providers are likely to try to act in an exemplary manner when being observed, which may not be their customary way of doing things. This means that direct observation tends to be more a measure of *maximal* performance than of *typical* performance, especially if it is done infrequently. If a measure of typical performance is desired, then it is probably advisable to observe the practitioner on multiple occasions. The subjects become used to being observed, and their behavior becomes more typical.

Record and Chart Review

Focused review of patient charts or other hospital records is the most commonly used technique for determining if participation in designated continuing-education programs results in changes in practitioner behaviors within their practice settings. Patient charts are the most frequently used data source. The type of information most commonly garnered from charts is frequency information — for example, number of services performed (McClellan and Cox, 1968), number of laboratory tests ordered (Foster and Lass, 1969; Rubenstein, 1973; McDonald, 1976), number of times a particular procedure is performed (Kane and Bailey, 1971; Talley, 1978), and number of times a particular drug or class of drugs is prescribed (Foster and Lass, 1969; Mock et al., 1970; Rubenstein, 1973; McDonald, 1976; Avorn and Soumerai, 1983; Rosser, 1983). Charts are also used to assess more complex behaviors — for example, drug-prescribing patterns (Bird, 1976; Laxdall et al., 1978; Rosser et al., 1981), diagnostic accuracy (DeBombal et al., 1974; Ashbaugh and McKean, 1976), quality of surgical care-related behaviors (Brown and Uhl, 1970; Devitt, 1973; Cayten et al., 1974; Devitt and Ironside, 1975), and quality of medical care-related behaviors (McGuire et al., 1964; Roney and Roark, 1967; Williamson et al., 1969; Reed et al., 1973; Grimm et al., 1975; Nelson, 1976; Payne et al., 1976; Harlan et al., 1980; Sibley et al., 1982; Gullion, et al, 1983). Examples of other types of hospital records used in evaluation of CE programs include laboratory records (Missouri Heart Assn., 1970; Eisenberg et al., 1977), pharmacy records (West et al., 1977), actual prescription slips (Manning et al., 1980), records of charges (Schroeder et al., 1973), and insurance-claim records (Buck and White, 1974; Brook and Williams, 1976). Patient charts are also the most commonly used source of information about changes in patient health status (Hirsch, 1974; Kattwinkel et al., 1979; Dickinson et al., 1981; Gullion et al., 1983), although use of other data sources is common, including use of epidemiologic data (Lewis and Hassanein, 1970; Reed et al., 1973).

Charts and records can be considered a type of product produced by the health-care provider. They provide a source of information about the quality of care provided across time. Further, the adequacy of the record itself is an important dimension of quality of care. As a product, their usage has the same basic advantages and limitations as any other product evaluation in comparison to a performance evaluation.

The first advantage is that the process of reviewing the chart or record is generally unobtrusive and done after the health care has been provided, thus avoiding the problem faced with direct observation, where the mere presence of the evaluator may alter the health-care performance. The second advantage is that the evaluators can review the charts or records at their own convenience. The same product can be reviewed by multiple reviewers to assess the reliability of the review instrument, without the necessity of all reviewers having to be in the same place at the same time. Further, in contrast to revision of an observational instrument, revision of the chart or record-review instrument does not necessitate locating new behavior samples.

The final advantage is that in general, product evaluations tend to be more reliable than performance evaluations.

The primary limitation of the use of charts and other records is that they provide only a partial and indirect picture of the actual care-related behaviors. For example, it is not possible to assess interpersonal skills using patient charts or hospital records. Another limitation is that records may be incomplete or inaccurate. Omissions in the record may indicate that appropriate care was not provided or it may be that the written record incompletely documented what was actually done.

It is important with the use of records, as with any other data source, that the information required to answer the research questions of the evaluation can be obtained from records. Further, specific predetermined criteria or standards should be prepared, against which the patient records can be compared. Finally, after the record-review instrument has been developed, the reviewers should be trained and the review process tested before the actual record or chart review begins.

One related approach to examining the process of health care merits special mention: the use of "tracers." This method, which involves chart review, is used in quality-of-care assessment and has the potential for use in evaluation of continuing education, particularly in major centers like the USC Development and Demonstration Center where more basic research on the effectiveness of CE is possible. A tracer is a specific diagnostic category or surgical procedure selected on the basis of six requirements: (1) it should have a definite impact; (2) it should be well defined and easy to diagnose; (3) rates of prevalence should be high enough to ensure an adequate sample of data; (4) natural history of the condition should vary with use and effectiveness of care; (5) management techniques should be well defined for at least one of the processes of prevention, diagnosis, treatment, or rehabilitation; and (6) effects of nonmedical factors on the tracer should be well understood (Kessner, 1973). Sample tracer variables include otitis media, iron deficiency anemia, urinary tract infection, essential hypertension, and cancer of cervix. After a tracer is selected, a thorough chart review on the designated patient sample is conducted, using clearly defined criteria.

Tracers have great potential for use in general assessment of quality of care where the level of care associated with the tracer is extrapolated to indicate overall quality of care for the designated facility or group of health-care providers. They also have potential for use in evaluation studies in CE. The first and perhaps most important use would be to help guide a focused needs assessment. Once tracer variables are selected and protocols designed, care related to the tracers would be examined for the target group of practitioners. Needs for CE could then be determined, instruction provided, and effectiveness assessed by a second review of care for the tracers. There is potential for enhancing the objectivity of measurement to the point where most of the review can be performed by nonphysicians.

Use of Multiple Measures

Use of multiple methods for data collection can add considerably to the scope of studies to evaluate the effectiveness of CE in the health professions. Use of multiple measures generally takes one of two basic forms: (1) combining methods to collect data on various levels of learning outcomes, i.e., learner satisfaction, knowledge/skills/attitudes, performance behaviors, or patient outcomes; or (2) using varied techniques to assess one outcome level, e.g., use of chart audit and self-report to assess changes in performance behaviors. The first method adds breadth to a study and allows analysis of the relationship among results at the different levels. The second method adds depth to the study of the effects of CE on one outcome level and enhances the likelihood of obtaining a reliable and valid picture of effects at that level. Clearly, combining these two forms in the same study will result in both increased scope of the levels examined and increased depth of analysis at selected levels. Use of multiple methods for data collection is always recommended where feasible. However, the choice of which methods, and at what levels, depends entirely on the objectives of the evaluation.

Evidence of the usefulness of multiple measures was presented by Stein (1981) in his examination of eight studies reporting significant results of the effectiveness of CE. He reported that all eight studies made use of multiple techniques for assessment with five studies collecting data on multiple levels (Buck and White, 1974; Condon, 1974; Laxdall et al., 1978; Talley, 1978; Kattwinkel et al., 1979), one using multiple measures to collect data on one level (Jewell and Schneiderman, 1978), and two studies doing both (Inui et al., 1976; Wang et al., 1979). In the other 40 studies included in my review, only 12 reported using multiple data-collection techniques.

Usefulness of *Standards* Relevant to Data Collection

This final section primarily summarizes the comments of Conference participants that are related to the *Standards* and data collection. Since Madaus provides a detailed discussion of each standard, it does not need to be repeated here.

Below is a summary of the Conference participants' comments about the overall usefulness of the 16 Standards relevant to data collection:

1. The participants basically agreed with Madaus's opening remark that the usefulness of any given Standard depends on the goals and scope of the proposed evaluation.

2. The participants felt that the *Standards* were designed for use primarily with large evaluations of lengthy educational programs serving captive audiences. Most CE programs are of short duration, with very small or nonexistent budgets for evaluation. Therefore, it is generally not feasible to consider the 16 data-collection Standards individually.

3. Participants did not quarrel with the need for data-collection Standards, but said that to be useful, the Standards must be tailored to the qualities and limitations of evaluation in CE.

4. Many participants felt that the *Standards*, even in their current form, might be a useful guide for those involved in large, well-funded evaluation studies.

The Conference participants also had the opportunity to discuss three of the Standards individually: C-5, Rights of Human Subjects; D-6, Reliable Measurement; and D-5, Valid Measurement. The participants felt that the Rights-of-Human-Subjects Standard raised important issues that need to be considered, especially when collecting data from patients. They felt, however, that the Standard, as written, had much less application when the data source is practitioners. In considering the Reliability and Validity Standards, the participants expressed real frustration with trying to meet these types of Standards in low-budget evaluations. They felt that often the best they could do was to assure careful preparation of all data-collection instruments. Preusage trial and statistical analysis to assess reliability or validity are generally not feasible.

The participants' overall reaction was that they were impressed with the need to develop and use standards for data collection, but quite overwhelmed with the volume and complexity of the set of Standards presented.

Summary

In this chapter I have attempted to accomplish three things: (1) to provide a critique of the Madaus discussion of issues related to data collection; (2) to supplement the Madaus chapter with a discussion of data-collection techniques used in evaluation of continuing education in the health professions; and (3) to summarize the comments of the Conference participants where appropriate. It is clear that the issues raised by Madaus are important ones to consider in all evaluation efforts, including those in CE. It is also clear that CE evaluators have many techniques available which can be used to gather useful information beyond participant satisfaction. One final thought: since most CE program evaluations must be done under severe time and fiscal constraints, CE evaluators might consider using several indirect measures for assessment, including a measure of behavioral change. Data collection and analysis for indirect techniques are relatively inexpensive and can provide a means of gathering behavioral data that should be feasible for all but the smallest programs.

References

Ashbaugh, D.G. and McKean, R.S. (1976). "Continuing medical education: The philosophy and use of audit." *Journal of the American Medical Association,* 236, 1485-1488.

Avorn, J. and Soumerai, S.B. (1983). "Improving drug-therapy decisions through educational outreach, a randomized controlled trial of academically based 'detailing.' " *New England Journal of Medicine,* 308 1457-1463.

Bacal, H.A. (1971). "Training in psychological medicine: An attempt to assess Tavistock Clinic seminars." *Psychiatry in Medicine,* 2, 13-22.

Bertram, D.A. and Brooks-Bertram, P.A. (1977). "The evaluation of continuing medical education: A literature review." *Health Education Monographs,* 5, 330-362.

Bird, W.A. (1976). *A Study of continuing dental education.* Thesis, Harvard University, Cambridge, Massachusetts.

Bloom, B.S. (1956). *Taxonomy of educational objective, Handbook 1: Cognitive domain.* New York: McKay.

Boeck, M.A. et al. (1972). "Continuing education: Assessment of value of discussion sessions and of course impact on physician practice." *Northwest Medicine,* 71, 519-522.

Brennan, J.G. et al. (1974). "Continuing education in alcoholism: Attitude change as a measure of seminar effectiveness." *Maryland State Medical Journal,* 23, 63-67.

Brook, R.H. and Williams, K.N. (1976). "Effect of medical care review on the use of injections: A study of the New Mexico Experimenal Medical Care Review Organization." *Annals of Internal Medicine,* 85, 509-515.

Brown, C.R. and Uhl, H.S.M., Jr. (1970). "Mandatory continuing education: Sense or nonsense." *Journal of the American Medical Association,* 213, 1660-1668.

Buck, C.R. and White, K.L. (1974). "Peer review: Impact of a system based on billing claims." *New England Journal of Medicine,* 291, 877-883.

Cameron, J.S. (1966). "Broadcast television for doctors — a first evaluation." *British Medical Journal,* 5492, 911-914.

Caplan, R.M. (1971). "Continuing medical education in your future." *Journal of the Iowa Medical Society,* 61, 207-212.

Caplan, R.M. (1973). "Measuring the effectiveness of continuing medical education." *Journal of Medical Education,* 48, 1150-1152.

Cayten, C.G. et al. (1974). "Surgical audit using predetermined weighted criteria." *Connecticut Medicine*, 38, 117–122.

Chambers, D.W. (1976). "How can learning experiences in continuing dental education be evaluated in relation to patient benefit?" *Journal of the American College of Dentists*, 43, 238–248.

Chambers, D.W. et al. (1976). "An investigation of behavior change in continuing dental education." *Journal of Dental Education*, 40, 546–551.

Condon, S.B.M. (1974). "Inservice education . . . impact on patient care." *Journal of Continuing Education in Nursing*, 5, 44–51.

DeBombal, F.T. et al. (1974). "Human and computer-aided diagnosis of abdominal pain: Further report with emphasis on performance of clinicians." *British Medical Journal*, 1, 376–380.

Devitt, J.E. (1973). "Does continuing medical education by peer review really work?" *Canadian Medical Association Journal*, 108, 1279–1281.

Devitt, J.E. and Ironside, M.R. (1975). "Can patient care audit change doctor performance?" *Journal of Medical Education*, 50, 1122–1123.

Dickinson, J.C. et al. (1981). "Improving hypertension control: Impact of computer feedback and physician education." *Medical Care*, 19, 843–854.

Donnelly, F.A. et al. (1972). "Evaluation of weekend seminars for physicians." *Journal of Medical Education*, 47, 184–187.

Driver, S.C. et al. (1972). "A comparison of three methods of using television for the continuing medical education of general practitioners." *British Journal of Medical Education*, 6, 246–252.

Durlack, J.A. and Burchard, J.A. (1977). "Preliminary evaluation of a hospital-based continuing education workshop on death and dying." *Journal of Medical Education*, 52, 423–424.

Edson, J.N. et al. (1969). "An evaluation of a clerkship in cardiology for general practitioners." *Journal of Medical Education*, 44, 1150–1155.

Eisenberg, J.M. et al. (1977). "Computer-based audit to detect and correct over-utilization of laboratory tests." *Medical Care*, 15, 915–921.

Forman, L.H. et al. (1964). "Evaluation of teaching efforts with nonpsychiatric medical practitioners." *Diseases of the Nervous System*, 25, 422–426.

Foster, J.T. and Lass, S.L. (1969). "A feasibility study using patient records to evaluate videotape postgraduate medical education (abstracted). *Journal of Medical Education*, 44, 980.

Garfin, L.A. (1969). "An evaluation of hospital dental seminars." *Northwest Dentistry*, 48, 167–168.

Gauvain, S. et al. (1965). "An experiment in postgraduate education to evaluate teaching and examination techniques." *Journal of Medical Education*, 40, 516–523.

Grimm, R.H. et al. (1975). "Evaluation of patient-care protocol use by various providers." *New England Journal of Medicine*, 292, 507–511.

Gullion, D.S. et al. (1983). "The effect of an individualized practice-based CME program on physician performance and patient outcomes." *Western Journal of Medicine*, 138, 582–588.

Harlan, W.R. et al. (1980). "Impact of an educational program on perinatal care practices." *Pediatrics*, 66, 893–899.

Hazlett, C.B. et al. (1973). "Evaluation of on-campus continuing medical education programs in Alberta." *Canadian Medical Association Journal*, 108, 1282–1287.

Hirsch, E.O. (1974). "Utilization review as a means of continuing education." *Medical Care*, 12, 358–362.

Holzemer, W.L. et al. (1980). "A program evaluation of four workshops designed to prepare nurse faculty in health assessment." *Journal of Nursing Education*, 19, 7–18.

Inui, R.S. et al. (1976). "Improved outcomes in hypertension after physician tutorials: A controlled trial." *Annals of Internal Medicine*, 84, 646–651.

Jewell, S.E. and Schneiderman, L.J. (1978). "Students in CME." *Journal of Medical Education*, 53, 1008–1009.

Jones, R., Jr. and Taxay, E.P. (1963). "Methodology and effectiveness of a program of postgraduate education for Cuban physicians." *Journal of Medical Education*, 38, 949–960.

Kane, R. and Bailey, R.Q. (1971). "Evaluation of a postgraduate educational programme in early cancer detection." *British Journal of Medical Education*, 5, 134–137.

Kattwinkel, J. et al. (1979). "Improving perinatal knowledge and care in the community hospital through a program of self-instruction. *Pediatrics*, 64, 451–458.

Kessner, D.M. et al. (1973). "Assessing health quality: The case for tracers." *New England Journal of Medicine*, 288, 189–194.

Laxdall, O.E. et al. (1978). "Improving physician performance by continuing medical education." *Canadian Medical Association Journal*, 118, 1051–1058.

Laxdall, O.E. (1982). "Needs assessment in continuing medical education: A practical guide." *Journal of Medical Education*, 57, 827–834.

Lewis, C.E. and Hassanein, R.S. (1970). "Continuing medical education — an epidemiological evaluation." *New England Journal of Medicine*, 282, 254–259.

Little, R.C. et al. (1983). "Change in obstetrician advice following a two-year community educational program on alcohol use and pregnancy." *American Journal of Obstetrics and Gynecology*, 146, 23–28.

Lloyd, J.S. and Abrahamson, S. (1979). "Effectiveness of continuing medical education: A review of the evidence." *Evaluation and the Health Professions*, 2, 251–280.

Lytton, B. et al. (1973). "Results of objective evaluation of postgraduate urologic seminar." *Journal of Urology*, 110, 582–584.

Mahan, J.M. et al. (1978). "Patient referrals: A behavioral outcome of continuing medical education." *Journal of Medical Education*, 53, 210–211.

Manning, P.R. et al. (1968). "Comparison of four teaching techniques: Programmed text, textbook, lecture-demonstration, and lecture-workshop." *Journal of Medical Education*, 43, 356–359.

Manning, P.R. et al. (1980). "Determining educational needs in the physician's office." *Journal of the American Medical Association*, 244, 1112–1115.

McClellan, T.E. and Cox, J.L. (1968). "Description and evaluation of dentist-dental assistant team training in efficient dental practice management." *Journal of the American Dental Association,* 76, 548-553.

McDonald, C.J. (1976). "Use of a computer to detect and respond to clinical events: Its effects on clinical behavior." *Annals of Internal Medicine,* 84, 162-167.

McGuire, C. et al. (1964). "Auscultatory skill: Gain and retention after intensive instruction." *Journal of Medical Education,* 39, 120-131.

Menzel, H.R. et al. (1966). "The effectiveness of the televised clinical science seminars of the New York Academy of Medicine." *Bulletin of the New York Academy of Medicine,* 42, 679-714.

Meyer, T.C. (1967). "Evaluation of the effectiveness of the telephone conference as a method of postgraduate education (abstracted)." *Journal of Medical Education,* 42, 874.

Miller, M.D. et al. (1978). *An innovative approach to home study correspondence courses in medical education.* Paper presented at the general meeting of the American Education Research Association Health Professions Education Special Interest Group, Toronto, Canada.

Missouri Heart Association. (1970). *Rheumatic fever and rheumatic heart disease: A terminal report of a detail man project.* St. Louis, Missouri.

Mock, R.L. et al. (1970). "Northern California postgraduate medical television: An evaluation." *Journal of Medical Education,* 45, 40-46.

Naftulin, D.H. and Ware, J.E., Jr. (1971). "Continuing education, clinical competence, and specialty certification." *Journal of Medical Education,* 46, 901-903.

Nelson, A.R. (1976). "Orphan data and the unclosed loop: Dilemma in PSRO and medical audit." *New England Journal of Medicine,* 295, 617-619.

Neu, H.C. and Howrey, S.P. (1975). "Testing the physician's knowledge of antibiotic use: Self-assessment and learning via videotape." *New England Journal of Medicine,* 293, 1291-1295.

Payne, B.C. et al. (1976). *The quality of medical care: Evaluation and improvement.* Chicago: Illinois: Hospital Research and Educational Trust.

Petersen, C.B. (1982). "An evaluation of the impact of a continuing education course in diabetes." *Evaluation and the Health Professions,* 5, 259-271.

Reed, D.E. et al. (1973). "Continuing education based on record audit in a community hospital." *Journal of Medical Education,* 48, 1152-1155.

Richardson, G.E. (1981). "A sexual workshop for health care professionals." *Evaluation and the Health Professions,* 4, 259-274.

Roney, J.G., Jr. and Roark, G.M. (1967). *Continuing education of physicians in Kansas: An exploratory end-result study.* Menlo Park, California: Stanford Research Institute.

Rosser, W.W. et al. (1981). "Improving benzodiazepine prescribing in family practice through review and education." *Canadian Medical Association Journal,* 124, 147-153.

Rosser, W.W. (1983). "Using the perception-reality gap to alter prescribing patterns." *Journal of Medical Education,* 58, 728-732.

Rubenstein, E. (1973). "Continuing medical education at Stanford: The Back-to-Medical-School program." *Journal of Medical Education,* 48, 911–918.

Schroeder, S.A. et al. (1973). "Use of laboratory tests and pharmaceuticals: Variation among physicians and effect of cost audit on subsequent use." *Journal of the American Medical Association,* 225, 969–973.

Shepherd, R.M. (1971). "Evaluation of continuing education." *Proceedings of the Royal Society of Medicine,* 64, 149–150.

Sibley, J.C. et al. (1982). "A randomized trial of continuing medical education." *New England Journal of Medicine,* 306, 511–515.

Stein, L.S. (1981). "The effectiveness of continuing medical education: Eight research reports." *Journal of Medical Education,* 56, 103–110.

Sula, J.A. et al. (1979). "Structured educational program for staff development." *American Journal of Hospital Pharmacy,* 36, 50–52.

Talley, R.C. (1978). "Effects of continuing medical education on practice problems." *Journal of Medical Education,* 53, 602–603.

Tucker, G.J. and Reinhardt, R.F. (1969). "Psychiatric attitudes of young physicians: II. The effects of postgraduate training and clinical practice." *American Journal of Psychiatry,* 126, 721–724.

Wang, V.L. et al. (1979). "Evaluation of continuing education for chronic obstructive pulmonary diseases." *Journal of Medical Education,* 54, 803–811.

West, S.K. et al. (1977). "Drug utilization review in an HMO: I. Introduction and examples of methodology." *Medical Care,* 15, 505–514.

Williamson, J.W. et al. (1967). "Continuing education and patient care research: Physician response to screening test results." *Journal of the American Medical Association,* 201, 938–942.

Williamson, J.W. et al. (1975). "Health accounting: An outcome-based system of quality assurance: Illustrative application to hypertension." *Bulletin of the New York Academy of Medicine,* 51, 727–738.

Woog, P. and Hyman, R.B. (1980). "Evaluating continuing education, a focus on the client." *Evaluation and the Health Professions,* 3, 171–190.

Worthen, B.R. and Sanders, J.R. (1973). *Educational evaluation: Theory and practice.* Worthington, Ohio: Charles A. Jones.

8 DATA ANALYSIS IN EVALUATION

William W. Cooley

One of the many nice things that the organizers of this Conference did was to prepare lists of questions on each of the topics for the four speakers. Unfortunately, when they arrived at the area of data analysis, they produced a very short list! At the top of an otherwise empty page was one item: "How can the evaluator best achieve the correct match between the data-analysis techniques and the quality of the data collected (i.e., how can we avoid using a cannon to kill a fly)?"

My immediate reaction was to wonder — how large a fly? Then I began to worry whether they were poking fun at my enthusiasm for canonical correlation a few years back. Upon a little more reflection, however, I decided that a more serious concern is that it is extremely difficult to address data-analysis problems in isolation of the total evaluation context. So I began to get a little sympathetic with the Conference organizers' not being able to give me a long list. That feeling of sympathy rapidly disappeared when I realized that the organizers are the same group that asked me to talk about this elusive topic!

So the next thing I did was to look at some background papers that were sent to speakers in preparation for this event. I thought I'd better become familiar with what this particular evaluation specialty has been doing. Most of the papers were concerned with the problem of establishing the impact of continuing-education activities in the health profession. After reviewing that set of papers it seemed most useful to address two different topics. One topic concerns analytic strategies, under the assumption that you are a researcher who wants to contribute to the knowledge about the effectiveness of continuing education in the health professions (CEHP). The other topic is client-orientation, under the assumption that you are an evaluator who wants to generate information that might inform current policy debates in CEHP, or produce information useful to a provider of CEHP that will help improve those services.

One topic I will not address is how you might serve a developer or provider of CEHP who wants you to do a summative impact study of his/her program. I have no solution to that untenable position. If you are successful in showing the impact of your boss's program, you lost your credibility with others; and if you're not successful, you lose your job! My only advice is to avoid such situations like the plague.

Experiments Versus Causal Modeling

Let me first turn to the problem of measuring program impact — attributing particular effects to particular CEHP treatments. To address the question of program impact, one must do everything that good researchers do or one will end up with hopelessly ambiguous findings. For example, you must be guided by the best available theory for the phenomena under investigation. That is, you have to have a good causal model for the factors known to be influencing the dependent variable(s) representing the expected outcomes of the CEHP treatment.

The causal model is essential if you want to guard against alternative explanations for what is producing the observed effects of the treatment. You must be well versed in the threats to both internal and external validity. That is, you must have good design, as Wolf pointed out.

Impact studies are evaluative in nature because the question of program impact is central to the question of the program's value. But in this context, the evaluator must do everything a good scientist does when supporting theoretical positions. Establishing a program's effects is clearly the most challenging research task an evaluator ever assumes.

One reason it is so difficult to establish a program's impact on a set of valued outcomes is that the experimental paradigm is almost never available in such field settings; furthermore, if tight experimental design is used as a device for obtaining credible internal validity, the constraints imposed by the experiment are so unlike anything that happens in "real life" that the generalizability of the findings are not credible.

One thing often lost sight of is that there has been so much emphasis on the importance of randomization of subjects to treatment that some other critical factors sometimes are ignored. For example, from what populations were the subjects drawn so as to provide a basis for generalizability? Even more important, how was the treatment level controlled so as to be sure that the experimental subjects did not participate in some "nonevent"?

Another remarkable thing that happens when people get all excited about their actually having done a randomized experiment is that they forget about statistical power. For example, in the experiment done by Sibley and associates (1982), in which they randomly assigned 16 doctors to two CEHP treatments, there is a real serious danger of Type-II error. They report accepting the null hypothesis that there is no difference in the quality of care provided between the treated and untreated doctors, but neglect to point out that even if there might be a real difference as large as a third of the standard deviation between the two groups of doctors, one would be accepting a null hypothesis 90 percent of the time that such an experiment was done with samples of that size.

But the main problem may have been Type-III error: testing the wrong hypothesis in the first place. For example, let's look at figure 8-1. This is a really simple (i.e., oversimplified) model of some of the factors involved in the 1982 experiment of Sibley and colleagues. They used quality of care as the dependent variable, had eight of the doctors use CME training packages, and left the other eight doctors to their own devices for gaining clinical knowledge that might, in turn, influence the quality of care they provide.

An observational study of the relationship between clinical knowledge and quality of care may have been more profitable. It is important to know what other factors influence quality of care besides clinical knowledge. There was some evidence that the CME packages were improving clinical knowledge, but the link between clinical knowledge and quality of care was too weak to show up as a significant difference between those who used the packages and those who did not.

Unfortunately, the dominant approach to assessing program impact has been to contrast experimental groups that receive the program and control groups that do not. The problems with this paradigm are many. Randomization is generally not available, and even if it is available initially, the type of longitudinal study that is required to estimate program impact results in high attrition which then presents other bias problems.

My own view is that we have a better chance of advancing the frontiers in estimating program impact if we work at it from the perspective of explana-

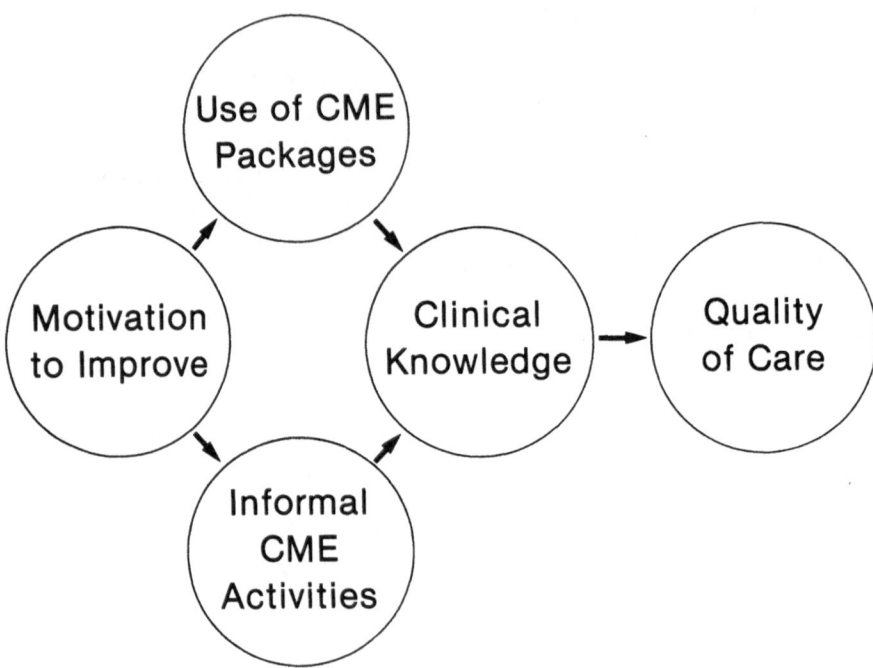

Figure 8-1.　Possible Causal Relations Among Constructs

tory observational studies (Cooley, 1978). In this mode, educational treatments are considered as multidimensional domains. The approach builds on what is being learned about causal modeling and causal inference. Any attempt to attribute educational outcomes to particular educational programs involves a causal model, whether it is implied by the procedures used or explicitly stated by the researchers. It is far better to make the model explicit and base the choice of statistical procedures on the model than to discover that the causal model employed is not a plausible model. People cannot be expected to accept estimates of the degree to which a program influences outcomes from analyses that are based upon nonbelievable models.

One problem with the state of the art in causal modeling is that the formulation of adequately specified models is way behind the development of statistical procedures that have been developed for evaluating their plausibility or estimating their parameters. The whole development of LISREL (Joreskog and Sorbom, 1979), together with the extensions that have been developed by Bentler (1980) and others, has produced rather impressive tools for studying causal models. The problem is that no one has done the tough scholarship required to review the literature of the phenomena under investigation and make sure that the major factors known to influence the dependent variables in an evaluation are taken into account as the investigator designs his or her study.

What seems to be forgotten is that a causal argument will be plausible to an audience only if they can't think of explanations (for the outcomes) that are alternatives to the explanation you are providing, and if their prior beliefs are not too strongly held, *and* if there isn't too much at stake. Whether a causal argument is plausible has very little to do with whether you did an experiment or an explanatory observational study.

Client Orientation

Let me turn now from the research task of establishing program impact to the way evaluation is facilitated by a strong client orientation. In this discussion, the context is a large urban school district, so you will have to make the transition to your field of CEHP.

In our school district work, we have set as our objective the generation of information which can be useful in a decision context, where the important decisions have to do with setting of priorities and allocation of resources. Our client orientation involves trying to understand the context in which the client makes decisions, identifying information which is missing in this context, then preparing data in ways that might inform those participating in the decision context (Cooley and Bickel, in press).

We have identified the school superintendent as our primary client. This is a little bit at variance with the "stakeholder" notion, but not as different as it seems. We do try to determine the perceptions of various people with a stake in the program being evaluated. It has proven to be very useful to contrast the perceptions of different groups and to compare those perceptions with other kinds of data. The problem is that *if* the evaluation activity is guided by the information requirements of a variety of stakeholders with a broad range of interests, the evaluation effort tends to try to serve everyone's needs for information and may very well end up serving no one very effectively. Our experiences have convinced us that it is essential to identify a *primary* client, and to serve that client well.

This client orientation includes trying to understand the client's need for information, involving extensive dialogue with the superintendent, both formal and informal, as well as observing him in interactions with the governing board and with the staff. It includes keeping notes of such meetings and organizing them in a way that allows one to trace a particular issue over time and establish what missing information might be helpful to the decision process. We also maintain a complete file of newspaper reports about school district issues and happenings so we can know what the public is being told about the district.

Client orientation does not mean doing the client's bidding. Rather, it takes the form of a mutual educational process. It requires a dialogue between client and evaluator out of which the needs for information are identified and strategies for obtaining it are defined. With respect to data analysis, the client-oriented evaluator must be methodologically eclectic. It is important to use the simplest statistical procedures possible so that the client can understand what has been done and why.

Another important feature of our work is how we try to get new information into the working knowledge of the participants in the decision context. (See Kennedy, 1982, for a good discussion of this notion.) This is as important as trying to figure out what information was missing in the first place. It is clear that busy managers do not read lengthy reports (Sproull and Larkey, 1979). Thus we have done our dissemination through interactive slide shows and informal conversations with the participants.

What is perhaps the most important emerging feature of our work is a shift from formal studies, which generally fall under the rubric of program evaluation, to a continuous activity of data collection and analysis, which I refer to as "monitoring and tailoring," the focus for the balance of my remarks.

Reform efforts in education have tended to assume that the best way to improve educational practice is to design and develop a new program which seems to address a particular problem, get schools to adopt and implement that innovative program, and then evaluate the program to determine its effectiveness in dealing with the problem. Berman (1980) calls this the technological-experimental paradigm of educational change. An alternative which has not been widely used in education and which has considerable promise involves developing and monitoring a variety of performance "indicators." Whenever an indicator moves into an unacceptable range, an attempt is made to determine why that condition exists. Then focused corrective action is taken which I call *tailoring*. On the surface it resembles the cybernetic model, but there are some very important differences. (Sproull and Zubrow, 1981, provide an excellent discussion of how the cybernetic model must be modified when applying it to an information system in education.)

Everyone is familiar with the thermostat, the classic example of the cybernetic model. The thermostat monitors an indicator of the temperature, and if the indicator moves into an unacceptable range, an action system is initiated automatically, adding heat if it is too cold and taking away heat if it is too hot: all very familiar. However, it is useful to review the thermostat analogy because it helps to see how a cybernetic model needs to be modified if it is to be successfully applied in education. Quite accurate devices have been developed for measurement of our physical world. Furthermore, it is quite feasible to establish an acceptable range of measurements for such indicators; and the relevant causal models are well developed, making clear what must be done if an indicator moves into an unacceptable range.

In applying the cybernetic model in education, it must be recognized that the available indicators are fallible, that it is not always clear what is an unacceptable range, and that it is not obvious what corrective action must be taken when an indicator moves into an unacceptable range. It certainly sounds almost hopeless. However, the monitoring and tailoring approach can be designed in ways which take these shortcomings into account and serve a very useful function within an educational system.

Our district-wide needs assessment is a useful illustration. One purpose of a monitoring and tailoring system is to help the district establish priorities for improving the system. Toward this end, we produced a variety of district-wide data which indicated the state of the educational system in the district. Briefly summarized, the indicators included (1) academic failures (25 percent of the students were failing ninth grade); suspensions (in a district of 45,000 students, there were 23,000); (3) class size (elementary school class size ranged from 10 to 32 students even for schools in adjacent attendance areas); (4) per-pupil costs (these were increasing much faster than the inflation rate over the past five years); (5) learning (one-fourth of the students leaving third grade were still not comprehending well enough to deal with fourth-grade curriculum, and 30 percent of the 11th graders were failing the minimum competency test in mathematics).

Extensive dialogue with the board of education regarding these and other indicators led the board to establish six priority areas for improving the educational program in the district. The dialogue not only was concerned with the degree to which the indicator was in an unacceptable range but also included discussions about which indicators pointed to more fundamental problems which, in turn, might be affecting the performance of other indicators.

The district-wide needs assessment (which includes both the data and the subsequent dialogue among board and superintendent) established that the most critical need in the district was to improve student achievement in the basic skills. Realizing that this was the most important concern, we analyzed all the available achievement data from the district, examining five-year trends, contrasts across grades, and differences among the various subject areas. The results of these analyses suggested that a major concern within achievement was reading in the primary grades. The data indicated that approximately 25% of the students were leaving third grade with reading comprehension skills inadequate to deal with the fourth-grade curriculum, not only in reading itself but in all subject areas. The district's previous reaction to the achievement slump that followed third grade had been to add and extend remedial efforts. By the sixth, seventh, and eighth grades, over half the students were in one or more remedial programs. We suggested a refocusing of efforts in the primary grades.

Further examination of the data (this time at the classroom level) revealed a few second- and third-grade teachers whose students were at the low end of reading growth. From the data, it appeared as though little or no reading growth was occurring in the course of the year for students placed in those teachers' classrooms. (Note that in this particular example the indicator is not end-of-year achievement level but *achievement growth*, and the units being monitored are classrooms, not students or schools.)

Now the question is, when it's discovered that a teacher's performance (as measured by the reading growth of that teacher's students) is in an undesirable range — what's to be done? Tailoring requires a deployable resource, which I call an "action system," that can respond to a performance indicator, showing a reading in an undesirable range. First of all, the action system must recognize that the indicator is fallible. What is needed is a procedure for confirming the indication. In this particular case, the person that responds to the indicator might be the instructional supervisor, trained in clinical supervision and capable of visiting that classroom, initially to confirm the indication that reading instruction is not going well in that classroom. If the indication is confirmed, the next step is to diagnose the situation and correct it through a program of intensive clinical supervision. If the effort of clinical supervision fails and is well documented, then there is an adequate basis for more drastic action.

One useful way to examine performance indicators is in their distribution. Noticing where unusually low performance is occurring on a priority indicator provides a basis for guiding the action-system which is supposed to improve that performance. The unit of analysis for examining distributions is the unit that is the focus of the action system. Classroom would be the unit of analysis for student-achievement data if the teacher is the focus of corrective action by a supervisor.

If district-level aggregates indicate that attendance has moved into an undesirable range, and the action system available for correcting truancy consists of social workers working with individual students and their families, then the distribution of student-level truancy rates would be examined for extreme cases. Similarly, if district-level aggregates indicate that student suspensions have reached an intolerable level, and the action system for dealing with excessive suspensions is a special team to assist the principal in re-establishing an orderly learning environment in that building, then the distribution of building-level suspension rates would be examined for extreme cases.

One assumption central to the monitoring and tailoring approach is that important, significant improvements can be made in the educational system through "fine-tuning" the system. There may indeed be some fundamental changes to be made in the system in order to adjust to fundmental changes that occur in society, but it does seem rational to make sure that current practices are working as well as possible before trying some dramatic departure from those current practices. I am not saying we should not innovate; in fact, I am calling for a kind of innovation. But some districts have tried to innovate too much and too readily. When a problem is detected, the tendency is to launch a district-wide solution, generally involving a new program, rather than determining exactly where things are not working well and tailoring practice to improve performance. The district-wide innovation can frequently disrupt things which have been working smoothly and seldom corrects situations that were not. Too little has been done to get the innovations working smoothly. But let's take a further look at some of the features of a monitoring and tailoring system.

First of all, it is important that multiple indicators are developed at multiple levels (i.e., student, classroom, school, and district levels). Since considerable information-processing would then be required, an essential ingredient is a computer-based information system to allow the development and display of the necessary indicators.

The required information system includes information on student programs and progress. With respect to student-level data, this would include information on student attendance, suspensions, curriculum, and test results. The computer file also indicates the sequence of teachers and school buildings to which each child has been assigned during his or her tenure in the district. These variables are then developed into indicators.

What is needed are indicators of two major constructs: (1) the degree to which the educational system is preparing its students for the future; and (2) the quality of the present experience. These constructs are generally reflected in indicators of student achievement and school climate. Dialogue regarding appropriate indicators of both constructs is extremely critical. Schooling is a large part of everyone's life. It is important to seek indicators of the richness of the present experience as well as satisfy the clamor for indicators of how well the students are being prepared for adulthood. (See Cooley and Lohnes, 1976, chapter 3, for further discussion of this important point.)

The continuous refinement and revision of the indicators is the primary task of the evaluator in such a system. One problem in using indicators is that it is frequently possible to corrupt them. That is, indicators are corruptible if it is possible to affect the indicator without affecting the underlying phenomena that the indicator is attempting to reflect. For example, if suspensions are being monitored as an indicator of school climate, and if having many of them reflects poorly on the principal, it is very easy to see how principals could modify their behavior with respect to issuing suspensions (or reporting them!) and still have the same actual level of trouble in that building. The corruptibility of indicators is one reason why it is important to have multiple indicators of the same construct and to refine them continuously. It should be pointed out that indicators will be corrupted more readily if rewards or punishments are associated with extreme values on a given indicator, than if the indicator is used for providing potentially corrective feedback.

Another requirement for monitoring and tailoring is to have the information system "connected" to an action system. *How* this is done is very important because it is usually not clear *why* an indicator shows values in an unacceptable range. Indicators are a function of the performance of a large number of factors in the system: students, teachers, principals, textbooks, supervisors, parents, central administration, policies, laws, etc. Monitoring indicators can tell you only where to look for possible problems. For that reason, the action system called into play must be, first and foremost, a diagnostic system. Corrective action is generally not clear from the indicators because our causal models for explaining their rise and fall are still not adequately specified.

The monitoring and tailoring approach requires the availability of services that can be deployed to correct the most serious cases found within the district. At the student level, dealing with extreme cases on such indicators as attendance, suspensions, and achievement growth might be social workers, counselors, and remedial tutors. Specialists trained in clinical supervision work with teachers who are outliers on classroom-level growth indicators; a school improvement team might work in schools that are extreme on building-level indicators.

I certainly hope you have found these remarks useful. I am not well enough informed about continuing education in the health professions to know whether or not the concepts of monitoring and tailoring are applicable, but I want to encourage you to examine them carefully. You may find it more useful in improving CEHP than little experiments which try to determine if doctors who are more knowledgeable about how to treat patients acually do provide higher quality care.

References

Bentler, P.M. (1980). "Multivariate analysis with latent variables: Causal modeling." *Annual Review of Psychology*, 31, 419–456.

Berman, P. (1980). *Toward an implementation paradigm of educational change.* Santa Monica, California: The Rand Corporation.

Cooley, W.W. (1978). "Explanatory observational studies." *Educational Researcher*, 7(9), 9–15.

Cooley, W.W. and Bickel, W.E. (1986). *Decision-Oriented Educational Research.* Boston: Kluwer-Nijhoff. In press.

Cooley, W.W. and Lohnes, P.R. (1976). *Evaluation research in education.* New York: Irvington Publishers.

Joreskog, K.G. and Sorbom, D. (1979). *Advances in factor analysis and structural equation models.* Cambridge, Massachusetts: Abt Associates.

Kennedy, M.M. (1982). *Working knowledge: And other essays.* Cambridge, Massachusetts: The Huron Institute.

Sibley, J.C., Sackett, D.L., Neufeld, V., Gerrard, B., Rudnick, K.V., and Fraser, W. (1982). "A randomized trial of continuing medical education." *New England Journal of Medicine*, 306(9), 511–514.

Sproull, L. and Larkey, P. (1979). "Managerial behavior and evaluator effectiveness." In H.C. Schulberg and J.M. Jerrell (eds.), *The evaluator and management.* Beverly Hills, Sage Publications.

Sproull, L. and Zubrow, D. (1981). "Performance information in school systems: Perspectives from organizational theory." *Education Administration Quarterly*, 17(3), 61–79.

9 ANOTHER VIEW OF DATA ANALYSIS

Kaaren I. Hoffman

Earlier in this Conference, Cooley indicated that to consider data analysis apart from the research questions being asked is very difficult. Certainly, throughout the course of the Conference, it was evident that analysis in and of itself was rarely criticized or even discussed — even when it was the assigned topic. Instead, criticism was addressed to the content of the research questions. Such an occurrence seems quite natural to me, for I have always sensed a certain amount of symbiosis between the research questions asked and the data-analysis methods used to answer them. Each seems to stimulate the other to new heights: as the questions become more comprehensive and complicated, new techniques are developed to answer them; and likewise, new developments in measurement and observational techniques allow new questions to be addressed.

This relationship between research questions and analytical methods can be most beneficial, but it does have its pitfalls. Shulman (1981) has pointed out that the various disciplines tend to ask different research questions based on their respective analytical perspectives, and he presents an intriguing account of how the various disciplines might approach research in reading. While such a strict discipline approach can be seen as too narrow, at least the questions and the methods are in accord. A greater danger, particularly in the area of evaluation, arises if the research question is actually redefined by the selection of the data-analytical procedures. In other words, the data-analysis techniques in the repertoire of an evaluator influence the type of questions that get answered, if not the type of questions that get asked. In their book on evaluation, Cooley and Lohnes (1976) present a perfect example of how data analysis frames or influences the evaluative question. Discussion centers on the analysis and subsequent reanalysis of data originally gathered by Coleman and others for the report "Equality of Educational Opportunity." Cooley and Lohnes point out that the original analysis due to selection of a step-wise regression procedure, answered the question, "What effect has schooling on achievement over and above effects of family and sociometric background?" However, in the reanalysis by Mayeske and associates, selection of the method of controlled variation resulted in answering the question, "What are the joint and unique effects of both schooling and family and sociometric background on achievement?"

In light of the foregoing, it is important to recap the discussion on the state of the art in data analysis in accord with the designated evaluational purpose or question. Cooley, in his presentation, has suggested that different analytical approaches are necessary for different evaluation purposes. I certainly concur, and the necessity of identifying the real purposes of the evaluation and delineating the intended use of the results was appreciated by the Conference participants as well.

Currently, there seem to be three distinct purposes or types of evaluation studies that parallel the evolutionary changes in the definition of evaluation itself (Nevo, 1983). The three types in reverse evolutionary order are (1) impact studies, (2) inquiry studies, and (3) instructional studies. The major trends in data analysis are different for each type of evaluation study; thus, each will be discussed separately.

Perhaps the greatest number of changes in data analysis have occurred in the newest type of evaluation: the impact study. As Cooley has pointed out, most of the evaluative studies within the impact arena are large-scale and rightly so. The research questions are multifaceted, and many different groups with vested interests are involved. The complexity and political nature of impact evaluation become apparent as one reads and notes the priorities in the *Standards* as well as in the other chapters presented in this book. Three major data-analysis trends can be delineated: (1) an increase in the complexity and multivariate nature of quantitative analysis; (2) an increase in attention to the reporting of the results (their reasonableness and their use); and (3) an increase in the use of and respect for qualitative analysis.

The area of impact evaluation is distinguished by its sophisticated quantitative techniques. The reciprocal relationship between the questions being asked and the techniques of analysis employed is particularly evident in this area. Complex questions have stimulated the application of multivariate analytical procedures, and the availability of multivariate procedures has encouraged the investigation of multifaceted issues.

Traditionally, educational evaluation studies of impact have employed multivariate correlational techniques such as path analysis, canonical correlation, and multiple regression. These techniques of controlled correlation are particularly adept at addressing the questions of mutual influence so common to impact evaluation (Cooley and Lohnes, 1976). Recently, several techniques for dealing with multiple latent (nondirectly measured) variables have reached new statistical manageability. This family of latent variable techniques include (1) the latent trait theories finding so many applications in the area of ability measurement (Traub and Wolfe, 1981); (2) the log-linear models applied to latent variables of a categorical nature (Bergan, 1983); and (3) confirmatory factor analysis and latent structural analysis applied to continuous variables (Joreskog and Sorbom, 1979). While these techniques differ on the type of latent variable they deal with, they all have in common the specification and subsequent testing of a model depicting the hypothesized direct and indirect relationships between the latent variables and their indicators and among the latent variables themselves. Such causal modeling, many believe, holds great promise for the area of impact evaluation where the establishment of influence patterns among relevant variables is often the major issue. Modeling ensures that the questions asked are carefully defined and patterns of interactions are detailed. However, as Cooley has stated, the latent variable techniques are quite complicated. Unique solutions are difficult to obtain even if one has the required statistical expertise.

In the area of health-professions continuing education, impact evaluation can be linked with what Houle (1980) has described as the estimation of the level of performance of an entire profession as made by its members, those serviced or the general public. There was considerable discussion at the Conference as to whether large-scale impact evaluations are currently being undertaken and/or even appropriate for the field of continuing education for health professionals. Certainly models specifying the variables involved in determining the effectiveness of continuing health-professional education will be of even greater complexity than those in general education. Links between health professionals' competence and recipients' health status are already indirect and weak, and these must be preceded by links between continuing-education practices and competence. Several other factors distinguish investigations into the impact of continuing education from those of general education. First is the fact that participants of continuing education are not a compulsory audience: they are not in attendance on a regular basis. Second, the providers of continuing education are for the most part not centrally organized (although certain associations and the Veterans Administration have such a potential). Finally, oftentimes the learning material, the case study or patient, is also the means by which results are measured.

The consensus of the Conference participants appeared to be that, regardless of whether the latent variable techniques were appropriate or whether they were engaged in large-scale impact studies, the exercise of modeling was seen as valuable. Participants believed that explicitly defining one's expectations as to treatment effects and specifying their direct or indirect nature would be of great benefit. Such specification clearly identifies areas in which additional or supplementary data analysis might be necessary and strengthens the overall data-analytic approach.

Clarifying one's expectations as to treatment effects can also be helpful when it comes time to report the results and specify the conclusions that can be legitimately drawn from the data. Thus, the second major development in data analysis pertinent to impact evaluation involves the current emphasis placed on the interpretability and usefulness of the results. Both the discussion of the *Standards* and Cooley's presentation have emphasized how important it is for the evaluator to identify the client of the impact study and to provide him with interpretable results. Judging from the *Standards*, a "science of change" has been superimposed on evaluation studies. Of particular note is the Standard of "justifiable conclusions." In many a sense, this Standard implies the legal standard of "beyond a reasonable doubt" where the consideration and comparison of all the evidence leave one able to say they have an abiding conviction of the truth of the matter. McCutcheon (1981) has done an excellent job of delineating the type of evidence and reasoning demanded of this Standard, and those involved in data analysis will find it interesting.

The desire to place practical value on the results has renewed interest in the more analytical topic of "effect size" or the determination of when treatment effects are to be considered of practical significance. A good review of the issues and the attempts to standardize effect size has been done recently by Sechrest and Yeaton (1982). A caution about considering practical effect size apart from statistical significance is well taken and has been noted by Hsu (1980) in response to Cohen's initial article (1979).

Part of the renewed interest in effect size has come about due to the application of meta-analysis techniques to a variety of areas. Meta-analysis, as discussed at the Conference by Cooley, is a statistical technique for integrating the existing research findings in an area. The methodology generated considerable interest among the Conference participants, seemingly related to the fact that so much of continuing education is decentralized. Many participants believed that much of their research or evaluation activities were too local to have widespread impact. Meta-analysis activity, however, seemed to hold the promise that their activities could be integrated with other findings to produce the desired impact. Whether this is true remains to be seen.

The two major trends in data analysis discussed so far, increased concern for the interpretability of results and increase in quantitative sophistication, seem directly related to the third and final trend — that involving the rise in qualitative analysis. First, it is important to recognize that quantitative information, while it perhaps offers proof, does not convince. McCutcheon's article (1981) mentioned earlier, as well as those by Eisner (1981) and Phillips (1981), have indicated how subjective information is still the prime mover of action. The complexity of some of the current quantitative techniques has perhaps strengthened this conviction.

The current use of qualitative data analysis, however, goes far beyond providing supplemental data designed to convince evaluation "clients." In recent years, one has seen the qualitative advocated in lieu of the experimental. A major thrust for this movement has been the belief that the problems being dealt with are too highly stochastic to afford any consistent quantitative predictive analyses. The major premise seems to be that descriptive analysis as well as other more qualitative analyses are more suited to such problems.

Interestingly, the same concerns resulting in an increase in the use of qualitative techniques have advanced the quantitative technique of exploratory data analysis (EDA). EDA (Velleman and Hoaglin, 1982) is perhaps best seen as an alternative approach to data analysis which proceeds step by step, variable by variable. While EDA is quantitative in format, its emphasis, similar to that of qualitative methods, is on gaining a thorough knowledge and understanding of the data, exceptions (roughs) as well as rules (smooths). It certainly seems more than coincidence that the popularity of EDA comes at a time in which high-speed computers have allowed the processing of complicated statistical procedures without the evaluator's ever having seen the raw data. EDA certainly gives one a "feel" for the data, similar to the feel one has when working with qualitative data. It stands as a unique technique with the great potential for hypothesis-generation as well as for hypothesis-testing. Oftentimes with EDA, the model follows from examination of the data rather than preceding it.

These, then, are what seem to be the major developments in data analysis in the area of impact evaluation: (1) an increase in complexity and modeling capabilities of quantitative analyses; (2) a similar increase and respect for qualitative analyses; and (3) greater attention to the interpretability and usefulness of the results of data analyses.

A wholly different approach to data-handling and -analysis can be seen within the second major area of evaluation, inquiry evaluation, epitomized as providing information for decision-making. Until recently, whenever an educational decision had to be made, a study was mounted to gather and analyze data specific to that decision. This procedure, as Cooley pointed out in his presentation, often led to incomplete or untimely results and disruption of current programs. Computerized longitudinal data bases, containing performance — as well as administrative — data, have the potential for revolutionizing the "crisis-oriented" studies so common in education. Cooley described a process of using these data bases he has called "monitoring and tailoring" which he has found exceedingly beneficial in his work with the Pittsburgh school district. In essence, monitoring and tailoring involves "getting ahead of the game," selecting data parameters to monitor, establishing acceptable boundaries for those parameters, and tailoring action and resources when a parameter crosses over a boundary. Obviously, such performance-monitoring involves the continual collection of, analysis of, and action from pertinent data.

Poister (1982) has noted the similarity and yet uniqueness of performance-monitoring to the more traditional administrative use of data bases termed process-monitoring which involves the tracking of resources going into a program and of outputs they produce. In describing his work with the Pennsylvania Department of Transportation, he proposes that performance-monitoring involves identifying (1) the program's objectives, (2) the logic underlying how the objectives are accomplished, (3) the performance indicators to be used for measuring progress, (4) the data sources from which measures can be drawn, and (5) the desired information flow of the results. Poister, like Cooley, was quite pleased with the usefulness of performance-monitoring in the area of decision-making evaluation.

The question now arises as to whether monitoring and tailoring is a feasible process for continuing education. A number of the participants expressed some doubt, finding it difficult to make the translation from a school system to the nonsystem and loose organization of providers of continuing education in the health professions. Others pointed to the Veterans Administration as an example of a system within the health profession area. Monitoring and tailoring does not seem to require the sophisticated system present in the nation's schools or even a system on the scale of the Veterans Administration to be either feasible or effective. All that is really necessary is an ongoing program of continuing education. Many such programs are probably already engaged in some degree of process-monitoring and hence require only the addition of "effectiveness data." Granted that effectiveness data are not easily gathered, the point is that difficulty in collecting such data is not an obstacle unique to performance-monitoring.

I see a major similarity between hospital or association-based "peer-appraisal" systems and the methodology of monitoring and tailoring. Houle (1980) has summarized some of the indispensable elements of hospital peer-appraisal systems, and I think the reader will find an obvious similarity between these features and those associated with monitoring and tailoring. On a larger scale, I would contend that the professional associations, with their measures of certification, recertification, and self-assessment, stand as a perfect example of repositories of continual performance data. Analysis of such data from a regional and/or a time basis would provide an excellent source of needs-assessment data, an area currently receiving considerable attention in continuing education (Houle, 1980).

On the whole, I find the technology of monitoring and tailoring to be very adaptable to continuing education. This is not meant to imply that the employment of such a system would be easy. The task of selecting effective indicators of performance and establishing appropriate standards is extremely difficult, particularly within professional health-care fields, due to the involvement of a third party — the patient. The effort, however, should be worth it, for in many respects the procedures demanded of continual performance-monitoring are more in line with the natural educational patterns of health professionals who learn as much or more from their work as from special organized programs (Houle, 1980). Finally, it should be noted that the creation of longitudinal data bases required for performance-monitoring are of value in and of themselves. Such data bases open the door for application of the techniques of time-series analysis (Ostrom, 1978) in which the impact of programs or natural events can be studied. In this manner, the procedures of monitoring and tailoring can be seen as effective for both inquiry and impact-evaluation studies.

I turn now to the final area of evaluation, that in which evaluation is seen as the process by which one ascertains if the objectives of a program have been met. This appears, judging by the discussions, to be the area in which the majority, or at least the vocal majority, of the participants are presently operating. Participants seemed to be primarily involved in the evaluation of instruction. I view instructional evaluation as the process of improving a pre-established instructional method or of ascertaining the generalizability of a particular method. Studies designed to compare one method of instruction with the other, I believe, are properly thought of as evaluation for decision-making or inquiry since the task itself assumes one has the option to select either of two different methods.

Three developments in the area of data analysis seem particularly pertinent to instructional evaluation. The first of them, determination of significant effect size, has been discussed previously under the area of impact evaluation. It is not uncommon for instructional-design experts to assume that if their treatment is good enough, large effects will be found. However, in the area of general education, the lack of large and consistent findings has already resulted in a redirection of research to an examination of aptitude-treatment interaction rather than treatment effects alone, and some believe even these research efforts will be bound by local considerations. Given the additional complexities of continuing education, the expectation of large treatment effects appears unreasonable and perhaps only achievable in the laboratory, if at all.

Effect size in instructional evaluation, just as in impact evaluation, needs to be put into perspective. As mentioned previously, the application of the thought processes of causal modeling techniques, if not the statistical techniques themselves, will contribute greatly to making explicit the actual connection between treatment and the measured outcome from that treatment. In reality, effects do not have to be either large or even significant for improvement to take place. In instructional design, evaluation should be considered an essential component of the process itself and, in analogy to the legal system, a criterion of the "weight of the evidence" should perhaps be used instead of "beyond a reasonable doubt." In other words, not as much evidence is needed to act on instructional improvements as would be needed for either impact or inquiry evaluation.

The second development in data analysis which probably will be of particular benefit to instructional evaluation is a statistical technique termed "matrix-sampling." Matrix-sampling is used for estimating the group mean on a performance measure without administering every item to every subject. For example, assume you had a 100-item performance test and a group of 200 participants. Normally, every participant would take the 100-item test. With matrix-sampling, the test is actually subdivided — perhaps into 10 subjects of 10 items each. These short subtests are then administered to subsamples of participants — for example consisting of 20 participants each. Studies have shown that a mean obtained through matrix-sampling procedures is as reliable, in terms of its standard error, as a mean obtained in the more traditional manner.

Matrix-sampling was originally formulated as a solution to several norming problems. However, it seems particularly valuable when applied to a pre- and post-instruction evaluation design. Although there are some restrictive assumptions, three advantages apparent for continuing education are (1) the saving of participant time, (2) the anonymity of individual response, and (3) elimination of potential biasing of results due to pretest sensitization. Documentation of the techniques of matrix-sampling can be found in Lord and Novick (1969).

While the use of matrix-sampling should ease the gathering of group data for instructional evaluation, the third and final relevant development of data analysis concentrates on the investigation of individual response patterns and involves a variety of techniques that can be grouped loosely under the rubric of "person fit techniques." In some respects, this development is similar to that of exploratory data analysis in that individual features of the data are seen to provide as much information as the group summary statistics; in part it is similar to the use of qualitative methods in that interest is as much centered on the *process* of learning as on the *product*.

Several techniques have been developed for analyzing person fit in regard to responses to educational achievement tests (Wright and Stone, 1979). In essence these procedures determine how internally consistent a person's responses (rights and wrongs) are and thereby how accurate or descriptive the summative measure (his overall score) is of his true behavior. The application of such procedures, with modifications, to instructional research might be extremely beneficial. Certainly the examination of individual behavioral or response consistency has previously been a neglected variable.

There is one more major development in education which, while it is not strictly within the data-analysis field, holds great promise for the area of instructional evaluation and continuing education in general. All of instructional research is starting to be influenced by findings within cognitive psychology which has placed emphasis on examining the process of mental activity or learning. Tobias (1982) has advanced the hypothesis that the manner (frequency and intensity) in which students cognitively process instructional inputs, and not the external characteristics of the instruction, determines the amount and/or type of achievement output. The idea of "meta-cognition," or the process of learning how to learn, should be of great interest to instructional design developers as well as planners of educational programs.

Another area of cognitive psychology that holds particular promise for continuing education is the examination of expertise and the structure, as apart from the amount, of knowledge. A good deal of the research, both theoretical and applied, in this area is pertinent to health professions education (Feltovich, 1983). Continual application of findings within these areas should contribute to new ways of looking at evaluation of program objectives in continuing education.

In summary, the trends in data analysis have in part been reflective of the major changes in the evaluation process itself as seen in the *Standards* as well as elsewhere. Data analysis, whether quantitative or qualitative, is far more diverse and eclectic in its application, with greater attention paid to the reporting, interpretation, and use of the conclusions arising from the analysis.

A number of the participants reported on the brevity of information provided for the data-analysis section in the *Standards*, expressing the desire for more examples and more references. The brevity is partly due to the technical nature of the subject matter, but also perhaps simply reflective of the priorities established by the Joint Committee in which utility, feasibility, and propriety are seen to precede accuracy. Such an ordering is in many respects natural and pertinent for the typical evaluative questions being addressed. Certainly within the area of impact evaluation utility, feasibility, and propriety are the major considerations.

The participants, for their part, echoed this feeling, for even when they had the specific task of performing a critique of an article's data analysis they overwhelmingly responded that the "wrong research question was asked." It is obvious that the appropriateness of the analysis was of secondary consideration. This subjugation of the technical aspects of analysis is, of course, appropriate, but it should not result in inattentiveness to the analysis procedures; for, as we have tried to elucidate, the selection of an analytic procedure can have a definite effect on the question actually answered. One must always be aware of this relationship and carefully inspect the analysis to determine if it in fact answers the question asked. In addition, the evaluator should consider a wide range of possible analytical procedures so as to make certain of the most powerful and appropriate selection in any given circumstance. The *Standards'* call for secondary analysis will be of great benefit, not necessarily to test any particular technique's restrictive assumptions but to delineate further the relationship among the questions asked, the data analysis, and the questions actually answered.

References

Bergan, J.R. (1983). "Latent class models in educational research." *Review of Research in Education*, 10, 305–360.

Cohen, J. and Hyman, J.S. (1979). "How come so many hypotheses in educational research are supported?" *Educational Researcher*, 8(11), 12–16.

Cooley, W.W. and Lohnes, P.R. (1976). *Evaluation research in education*. New York: Irvington Publishers Inc.

Eisner, E.W. (1981). "On the differences between scientific and artistic approaches to qualitative research." *Educational Researcher*, 10(4), 5–9.

Feltovich, P.J. (1983). "Expertise: Reorganizing and refining knowledge for use." *Professions Education Researcher Notes*, 4(3).

Houle, C.O. (1980). *Continuing learning in the professions.* San Francisco: Jossey-Bass Inc.

Hsu, L.M. (1980). "On why many hypotheses in educational research are supported and on the interpretation of sample effect sizes: A comment." *Educational Researcher*, 9(5), 6-10.

The Joint Committee on Standards for Educational Evaluation. (1981). *Standards for evaluations of educational programs, projects, and materials.* New York: McGraw Hill.

Joreskog, K.G., and Sorbom, D. (1979). *Advances in factor analysis and structural equation models.* Cambridge, Massachusetts: Abt Associates.

Lord, F.M. and Novick, M.R. (1969). *Statistical theories of mental test scores.* Reading, Massachusetts: Addison-Wesley.

McCutcheon, G. (1981). "On the interpretation of classroom observations." *Educational Researcher*, 10(5), 5-10.

Nevo, D. (1983). "The conceptualization of educational evaluation: An analytical review of the literature." *Review of Educational Research*, 53(1), 117-128.

Ostrom, C.W., Jr. (1978). *Time series analysis: Regression techniques.* Beverly Hills: Sage Publications Inc.

Phillips, D.C. (1981). "Toward an evaluation of the experiment in educational contexts." *Educational Researcher*, 10(6), 13-20.

Poister, T.H. (1982). "Performance monitoring in the evaluation process." *Evaluation Review*, 6(5), 601-623.

Sechrest, L. and Yeaton, W.H. (1982). "Magnitudes of experimental effects in social science research." *Evaluation Review*, 6(5), 579-600.

Shulman, L.S. (1981). "Disciplines of inquiry in education: An overview." *Educational Researcher*, 10(6), 5-12.

Traub, R.E. and Wolfe, R.G. (1981). "Latent trait theories and the assessment of educational achievement." *Review of Research in Education*, 9, 377-435.

Tobias, S. (1982). "When do instructional methods make a difference." *Educational Researcher*, 11(4), 4-9.

Velleman, P.F. and Hoaglin, D. (1981). *Applications, basics, and computing of exploratory data analysis.* Boston, Massachusetts: PWS Publishers.

Wright, B.D. and Stone, M.H. (1979). *Best test design.* Chicago, Illinois: Mesa Press.

10 POLITICS OF EVALUATION

Stephen Abrahamson

Considering the academic ideals and scientific principles involved in sound evaluation practices, one must wonder about the inclusion of a chapter on politics of evaluation in a major conference on evaluation of continuing education for health professionals. That is, by what reasoning did the planners of this Conference decide to include a discussion of politics when the other major topics so neatly and logically addressed truly central aspects of evaluation: problems of design, of data collection, and of data analysis?

The University of Southern California's (USC) Conference Planning Committee, interestingly enough, did have a logical basis for its decision to include such a presentation and a workshop discussion session in this three-day Conference. In its original deliberations, as the group began to discuss possible needs for such a conference, the faculty in the Department of Medical Education and other evaluators working on continuing education projects in the Development and Demonstration Center in Continuing Education for Health Professionals were asked to indicate problems they had encountered in conducting educational evaluation studies. That list of problems became the basis for selection of topics for this Conference.

Nine of those problems seemed to be concerned with nontechnical questions and involved, instead, questions of management, of decision-making, and of reporting practices. At first the Conference Planning Committee was inclined to create a category of "administration" to join those of design, data collection, and data analysis. But it was clear that much more than administration was involved; indeed, simple administration was perceived to do the nine problems a disservice. So this topic became the chapter you see today: "Politics of Evaluation."

If the often-bitter truth were known, there are no problems in the political arenas of evaluation that I have not experienced; after all, I have been here at USC as Director of the Division of Research in Medical Education for 20 years. During that time, we have conducted and participated in evaluation studies large and small, simple and complex, expensive and cheap (indeed, all-too-often, free), sophisticated and naive. There cannot be one mistake that we have not made at least once during those 20 years — mistake, that is, in the *political* arena. Generally, we have maintained high quality over the years. But when it came to operating politically, we frequently found no precedent and no role model to help us. After all, 20 years ago in continuing medical education it was considered innovative — nay, even radical — to attempt a simple cognitive test before and after a continuing-education program. I can recall 17 years ago using a 50-item multiple-choice test at the end of a five-day program for chest physicians and overhearing one participant mutter, "This is just the sort of goddam thing USC people would do!!"

Simply enough, then, my intent here today is to bring those 20 years of experience to bear in examining evaluation problems which have a political base. Essentially, my approach includes (1) describing political problems and their sources, (2) concentrating attention on conflicts, (3) sharing my views of management of problems of this kind, and (4) bringing you Abrahamson's view of the state of the art.

Problems and Their Sources

Of the many dictionary definitions of *politic*, I particularly like Webster's three definitions because of their relevance to our discussion: (1) "characterized by shrewdness," (2) "sagacious in promoting a policy," (3) "shrewdly tactful." These are particularly appropriate because it seems to me that politics in this context really refers to a set of personal techniques of management of evaluation. An evaluator is "good," therefore, in the politics of evaluation when he or she is shrewd, sagacious, and/or tactful. Politics, in sum, is the strategy and tactics of solving problems associated with evaluation.

These problems are difficult to separate from their sources; thus, the next section treats both the sources and problems which arise from them.

Maintaining evaluation standards represents a set of activities which all good evaluators would consider "part of the job." The earlier speakers have offered us all a panoply of suggestions, advice, and counsel all to the point of improving the quality of program evaluation. When one tries to do that, however, problems arise. Who should make decisions about evaluation study design, for instance? Can such decision-making be left with the program director? How much power can be delegated to the evaluator? The same questions, of course, apply to field techniques and to analysis of data as well as to study design. In our honest concern for our professional activities in evaluation, in our zeal to maintain standards, we will encounter problems.

Applying evaluation principles, like maintaining evaluation standards, is a source of problems. (Imagine: just trying to do our job becomes a source of problems!) For instance, what do we do with evaluation data that are apparently unfavorable to the interests of the program planners? This problem lies in wait for all of us any time we are engaged in evaluation activities. After all, one cannot be sure at the outset that the data will show *any* program achievement, let alone the hypothesized gain, for a given educational effort. But more than that, data other than those directly answering the major evaluation question might emerge. If they are unpleasant, are they then to be hidden? In one study, for instance, many years ago, we discovered some vital information. We were attempting to ascertain whether a certain slide-tape program had been successful in promoting learning among a sample of health professionals. We discovered that there was no significant learning gain — but, more than that, we also discovered that many of the health professionals (the "subjects") had not even seen the slides or heard the tapes. Good principles of evaluation suggest that the new information be included in the report. The program director, however, fearful that such information might strike the death knell to his total program efforts, ordered those data to be omitted. A problem? You bet.

Reaching agreement, a simple matter in many instances, can become a major source of problems. Here I refer to agreement concerning the processes of evaluation. What is the "best" time for the evaluator to begin her/his work? How do we determine the optimum cost-benefit ratio in evaluation design? If we leave that question to the evaluator, costs may be high; if we leave that question to the program sponsor, costs are probably low. Absurdity seems to appear when an estimate of the cost of evaluation is as high as the estimate for conducting the program to be evaluated. Of course, that might not be so absurd if the sponsors were considering the expenditure of millions of dollars in replicating the educational program. Then, of course, one might want the "best" evaluation, no matter what the cost. We found absurdity to be more frequent at the other end of the continuum. We were once asked to be "outside evaluators" on a million-dollar educational effort involving 60 educational packages to be used in 65 hospitals — and discovered the entire amount of money set aside for evaluation to be $5,000!

Obtaining compliance, a frequently necessary part of evaluation activities, is still one more source of problems. Not only are we faced with the problem of subjects who decline (refuse) to complete data-collection forms but we have internal problems as well. For instance, how do we get the program director (or other program staff) to use the evaluator appropriately? Considering the fact that evaluators see for themselves a significant role, what can be done to ensure that others see that same role — and use it to the advantage of the total effort?

Conflicts

The more one reviews sources of problems and the kind of problems they seem to generate, the more one begins to see problems as expressions of *conflict.*

Some are conflicts of values. Surely the example above — of a sponsor willing to spend a million dollars on an educational program but only $5,000 on its evaluation — is a statement of values. But it is then a conflict in values between that sponsor and the evaluator — perhaps even between that sponsor and the program director. Moreover, consider this experience we had some years ago. We had been retained to "evaluate" a major educational effort in continuing medical education. We were so bold as to believe that we should look at changes in physician behavior (practices) *since the objectives of the program were stated in those terms.* The program director stated that he believed the program would not bring about those changes and told us, instead, to limit our efforts to measuring only what he believed might show "gain." The conflict seems to be over what to measure, when in fact it is a value conflict and, therefore, much more complex to understand and much more difficult to manage. That is, while the disagreement was over what to measure, the conflict lay in the value of showing some success versus the value of integrity of evaluation design.

Closely related to value conflicts are those which arise from the impact of competing *vested interests.* One of our early debacles featured a series of improbable confrontations about almost every aspect of the program evaluation: design, data collection, data analysis, and finally, even reporting. On the surface it seemed that the project director, the sponsor, and the evaluator were simply disagreeing about each of these technical points of the evaluation. These disagreements, however, were but the surface manifestations of far deeper conflict. The project director and his staff had a vested interest in the program and were continually trying to increase the monetary base for their total efforts. The sponsor — a government agency — was engaged in a massive effort to accumulate evaluative data which would show that their government "mission" was being successfully accomplished — and the sponsor didn't care how that was achieved! The evaluator, like all of us who toil in this corner of the Lord's vineyard, wanted to maintain quality in order to enhance the reputation of his evaluation group. Once we all realized that we were not quarreling over the design, the data collection, and the reporting, once we realized that we were each zealously guarding our respective vested interests, then we were able to resolve our bitter problems and move to the tasks at hand. Of course, at that magic moment, the damned project was completed! That is, in the words of the old adage: we get so soon old and so late smart. An earlier recognition of the true nature of our conflict would have been enormously beneficial to all of us — and particularly to the program evaluation.

Finally, and again closely related to the conflicts described above, we have conflicts which derive from the pursuit of *personal goals.* In one evaluation project, for example, we had to try to deal with a project director who dictated design changes in the middle of the evaluation. At first, we treated it as if it were a simple expression of the director's conviction that he knew better than the evaluator what should be done at the particular moment — or "point in time," as one nefarious crew was wont to say. What we discovered as we attempted to deal with this curious intrusion was that the project director had found a way to make him look better and simply was putting pressure on the evaluation staff to do so. In this case, we made the discovery early enough to be able to avert disaster, but it wasn't easy. All we had to do was convince the director that the changes he was proposing would probably eventuate in his looking worse, not better. And that was difficult because his suggestions, in fact, would have made him look good.

Another illustration comes to mind because it was so bizarre and also because it hurt so much. We were conducting an evaluation study for a group that had a six-person executive committee. The chairman of that executive committee was the person who had initiated the contract between his organization and our evaluation group; he was also the person who had obtained the financial support for the effort. He seemed to us to be a leader, a charmer, a well-liked person. The six-person group knew each other well and drank well together; they shared many light moments both informally and during work sessions. But every time we delivered a progress report or conducted a work session to obtain their counsel, we found ourselves verbally flayed by one, several, or all of the six. Our debriefing sessions could not seem to help us: our work was good; our movement toward goals was exceeding expectations; our interpersonal relationships were warm. Yet, we seemed always to be in trouble. We embarked on a carefully conceived little program of data collection on our processes: observation, conversation, and speculation with validation. What we discovered — unfortunately late in the project, but still within time for potential rescue — was a mess caused by conflict growing out of personal goals totally irrelevant to the project. Simply stated: three of the five members of that executive committee wanted to be chairman; four of the five thought the chairman of that time was inadequate; the chairman thought he was doing a great job; and none of this was overt! The evaluation team was serving as the most marvelous whipping boy ever! It didn't matter what the topic was, what the tasks were, what the achievements were; we were soon defending ourselves from attacks on one side or another. There was one incredible session which occurred shortly after we had made our great discovery. Realizing that we were destined to be in the middle because of the committee members' personal goals, we carefully selected the one member who was most objective, apparently uninvolved in the political morass of that group, to give us the first reaction to a new data-collection device we had just designed. He had already tested it, and we knew he liked it very much. So, at the progress-report meeting, I casually turned to him and said, "Why don't you give us your reaction first, just to start our discussion?" (Obviously, getting a positive reaction at the outset was far more likely to beget a constructive discussion and a useful revision of the device.) His response will live with me forever: "The more I've thought about it, the more worried I am about it." Unbeknownst to us, one of the other executive committee members had "reached" him just before the meeting and had convinced him of the necessity to express serious reservations about these next steps. But those "reservations" were not substantive; they were purely political.

Context for the State of the Art

At this point, we may be ready to consider the state of the art. Sources of problems and the problems themselves have been discussed, with particular emphasis on conflicts — of values, of vested interests, and involving personal goals. In an effort to place that state-of-the-art review in a useful context, I would like to remind you that this Conference is taking place in California, the state that has given the nation a song-and-dance man for senator and a movie actor for president. Since we are in the motion-picture capital of the world, what better way to consider the state of the art than to put it into the context of cinema: the "Art of the State."

Like a cinematic production, the politics of evaluation has five major components: plot, cast, setting, scenario, and script. The *plot elements* include the familiar four: evaluation design, data collection, data analysis, and reporting. It is in the effort to get the work finished that our political problems arise. As we go about the complex and technically challenging tasks of designing the evaluation research, of collecting the necessary information, of analyzing and interpreting those facts, and of preparing a report describing the project, its evaluation, and recommendations relevant and appropriate to the evaluation, all of the cast of characters are involved. Therefore, since interactions among people are involved, problems may result.

The *cast of characters* includes (1) the sponsor, (2) the project director, (3) the evaluator, (4) the project staff, and (5) the subjects (dare we call them "extras"?). The sponsor, of course, is the person (or group) funding the educational effort and its evaluation. Obviously, the sponsor has a major interest in the project and often is the person (or group) most concerned with sound evaluation. The sponsor *should* want to know whether the project is successful: it is his (or their) money that is supporting the whole effort.

The project director is the person responsible for the conduct of the continuing-education effort. That effort may be a course, a lecture, a conference, a residency, a fellowship, a slide-tape package, a videotape package. Obviously there are many forms of project which may require evaluation. But there is always a director. There may be times when the director is also the sponsor. That would be true, for instance, in the case of a unit (department, division, bureau) of continuing education which conducts a program without outside support (other than tuition fees paid by participants). In that case, one would expect a minimum of conflict between the sponsor and the director. Notice the use of the expression, "*minimum of conflict.*" Even though the two characters are portrayed by the same person, the function of role is such that he or she could still find himself or herself in a kind of Hamlet-of-continuing-education role.

The third member of our cast of characters is the evaluator. It is not by chance that she or he appears in the middle of this listing. The nature of the work places her or him squarely in the middle much of the time. Through her specialty training — formal or on-the-job — she has acquired a set of skills and the necessary supporting sciences to enable her to answer crucially important questions and thus influence the very professional lives of the sponsor and the project director. Moreover, she or he also quite directly influences the lives of the other two members of the cast of characters: the staff of the project and the subjects included in the data collection.

Sometimes the staff of a project — particularly those involved in evaluation activities — place pressure on the evaluator to "maintain standards"

Table 10-1. Roots of Trouble

| | Plot Elements | | | |
Cast of Characters	Design	Data Collection	Analysis	Reporting
Sponsor	X	0	0	X
Director	XX	X	0	XX
Evaluator	XX	XX	XX	XX
Staff	XX	XX	XX	X
Subjects	0	XX	0	0

or "apply principles" and thus force the evaluator into conflict with the project director or even with the subjects from whom data are to be collected.

Briefly, the remaining three components are the *setting,* which is the project to be evaluated; the *scenario,* which is the problem situation posed to the evaluator; and the *script,* which is the management of that problem. These problems can range from simple to complex, from easy to difficult, from purely technical to highly personal. The matrix displayed in table 10-1 presents a graphic representation of sources of conflict.

Problems can occur at any point at which two or more of the cast of characters are involved in any one of the plot elements. And since good evaluation demands involvement by most of the cast in almost all of the plot elements, it is hardly a wonder that conflict arises and presents a problem. The double-checked entries represent essential involvement; the single

Table 10-2. Components of Politics of Evaluation

Plot (Elements)

Evaluation design
Data collection
Data analysis
Reporting

Cast of Characters

Sponsor
Project director
Evaluator
Project staff
Subjects

Setting = the project
Scenario = the "problem situation"
Script = the "problem management"

check, desirable involvement; the zero, contraindicated involvement. Unfortunately, contraindicated involvement frequently appears, bringing with it aggravated problem conditions.

By way of summary, table 10-2 reviews the components of the politics of evaluation.

Management of Problems

Just as the practice of medicine is divisible into two major categories, preventive and curative, the management of problems in evaluation of continuing education — the politics of evaluation, if you will — can be considered in the same two classes of action. Prevention of occurrence of problems may not always be possible, but certain actions *before* problems can occur will minimize their damage, if not avoid their emergence. Other actions may alleviate the situation *after* the problem appears.

Before problems occur, of course, is the best time to take action since the prevention or minimizing of problems makes the conduct of the difficult and complex task of evaluation that much more manageable. There are four suggestions here, based on our experience, particularly our experience in having failed to do these things!

1. *Anticipate your problems.* The first step in fruitful anticipation is to remember that the person who stated Murphy's Law ("if anything can possibly go wrong, it will") was an optimist! A good evaluator lists all the things that can possibly go wrong and begins to think about how to avoid them. The evaluator should try a careful analysis of the other members of the cast of characters. Who has what to gain? Who has what axe to grind? What are the hidden agendas? What different ego needs are manifest? Unfortunately, training in educational evaluation does not include developing skills for tasks of this kind. Yet, success of an evaluation effort may well depend on such careful assessment — and administrative steps to minimize potential damage.

2. *Establish standard operating procedures* (SOP). All too often problems appear or are exacerbated because of the lack of SOP or simple ground rules. Like the last three lines of that famous old limerick, "They argued all night/Over who had the right/To do what and with which to whom," failing to delineate ahead of time lines of authority and responsibility, neglecting to describe clearly what tasks need to be done, omitting reference to who makes what decisions can lead to endless argument and — worse than that — major obstacles to completing the evaluation. List all the tasks that must be done; draw a table of organization with lines of authority and responsibility; show

all the decision points, but then add a second level of detail: who is supposed to do each of the tasks, who is in charge of what, who participates in which of the decisions. And don't be embarrassed to write these things out in detail. So many of the errors described earlier in this chapter could have been avoided with such simple steps as these.

3. *Describe grievance procedures.* Remember Chisholm's corollary to Murphy's Law: "If *nothing* can possibly go wrong, it will anyway." Despite your best efforts to prevent problems, there will be some that occur. Many of these will be interpersonal problems. Indeed, even in the preventive actions of making those lists, conflict may arise. Any person functioning in a situation that permits disagreement may perceive himself or herself to be aggrieved. How can such a person appeal? Who is the final arbiter? Here, we are not referring to "settling things" before the work gets started; rather, we are trying to establish the procedures by which someone who feels aggrieved in the middle of the project can take steps to resolve issues, disagreements, conflicts. There might be a section of the evaluation protocol which states quite simply, "In case of disagreement, the following actions should be taken."

4. *Use mediation procedures.* Even during the earliest stages of planning the evaluation, perhaps even during recruitment and hiring of staff, disagreements can emerge. Using good mediation can be helpful in more ways than just resolving the immediate situation. Obviously, if two or more characters are in conflict or disagreement, mediation can help to solve that conflict or disagreement. More than that, sound mediation can help to establish both an atmosphere of cooperative activity and a technique for solving future problems.

Despite the best efforts at preventing problems, it is clear that some problems will occur anyway. Thus, one needs strategy for management when they do arise.

After problems occur, all is not necessarily lost. Here are another four suggestions — again, based on experience.

1. *Use diplomacy.* Unfortunately, this seems to be becoming a lost art. At the international level, confrontation, bluff, threat, and, all-too-often, warfare have emerged as the modern-day modus operandi. But the old-fashioned way — tact, diplomacy — still has much to offer. Conciliatory gestures, soothing phrases, genuine search for fault in oneself, tactful responses, all can help in relieving the tension associated with problems, thus making it easier for solutions to be found. Sometimes, gaining respect can come more constructively and more easily through diplomacy than through "winning" an argument.

2. *Compromise.* Of course, in a sense, this suggestion might be considered part of diplomacy. But it is important enough to mention by itself. Sometimes we become so convinced that we are right, that we insist — "as a matter of principle" — when it is evident to any objective outsider that the same result (desired by the evaluator) might be achieved with some "give" by that person.

3. *Use arbitration.* Part of the establishment of ground rules or SOP should include careful delineation of who has the "final say." More than that, it probably should also include procedure by which even an outside person might be the "court of last resort" for an impasse over evaluation procedures. That is, sometimes it is possible to establish as part of the ground rules that when an impasse occurs, a certain consultant will be asked to review the matter and recommend (mandate) a resolution to the disagreement.

4. *Surrender.* There is no question that the evaluator is by conventional structure the third most powerful person (or agency) within a project. Unfortunately for her or him, the most powerful person is the sponsor and the second most powerful, the project director. (Sometimes these two hierarchical positions may be reversed, but the evaluator still is number three!) A shrewd evaluator knows when it is time to yield, to give up. Furthermore, there are occasional concessions that can be elicited when one surrenders. But the caution here is that one should *not* try to exact anything in return. The true affect should be one of the old adage, "When it is inevitable, relax and enjoy it."

A quick comparison of the two lists of suggestions reveals one very interesting difference. Included among the suggestions for *before the fact* is *mediation;* among the *after-the-fact* suggestions is *arbitration.* Our view is that before problems occur, one can discuss things more easily, and mediation — with or without a mediator — can be quite successful and can produce those secondary gains alluded to above. But once the problem has occurred, it is probably no longer feasible to devote time and energy to that process — particularly when the problem involves sharp disagreement (an "impasse" is the way it is worded above) and also when quick action is needed to keep things moving.

It is also interesting to note that the "suggestions" are all outside the world of evaluation! That is, they do not demand skills in evaluation; they do not demand a knowledge of evaluation; they are skills of human relations, of interpersonal communication. However, the education and training of evaluators do not include learning experiences designed to make them skillful in these areas. Yet, I would hypothesize that more evaluations fail because of inability to resolve political problems than because of lack of technical knowledge and skill on the part of the evaluator.

State of the Art

What can now be said about the state of the art? To this point we have established certain conditions, definitions, and principles associated with political aspects of evaluation. These might well be reviewed as a start.

Recapitulation

Politics, in the context of this chapter, is really techniques of management employed by those involved in the evaluation process. And these are quite personal, undoubtedly idiosyncratic. Furthermore, in my definition is the notion that politics includes the strategy and tactics of solving problems.

The problems seem to arise from the natural, orderly process of "doing one's job." That is, they come from attempting to maintain evaluation standards, apply evaluation principles, achieve agreement, and obtain compliance.

Resolution of conflict is the most important part of the politics of evaluation. Conflicts appear between and among the members of the cast of characters: the sponsor, the director, the evaluator, the staff, and the subjects — all of whom want to (and should) participate in the decision-making concerning the processes of evaluation: design, data collection, analysis, and reporting.

But resolution of conflict may not be necessary if conflict is avoided. Thus, there are preventive steps that might be taken *before* problems arise as well as corrective measures *after* they occur.

The "True" State of the Art

Considering the fact that one becomes political in order to solve non-technical problems, it should not come as a major surprise to discover that the state of the art in politics of educational evaluation is essentially the state of the art in human relationships. In our settings, the state of the art is only as good as the management we are able to use *before* there are major problems, conflicts, or confrontations. (Some refer to this as "proactive.") So we are really talking about strategy. Unfortunately, the best teacher to date has been experience. However, it would be tragic if each of us had to have each bad experience (at least once) in order to develop skills of management which might facilitate our work.

One can find some help in the *Standards* which we have been considering during this Conference. These standards are derived from the experience of others. Careful consideration of what is included there can lead us toward state-of-the-art management of political events.

It is quite clear that evaluators — like automobile drivers — must anticipate and plan defensively. It is too bad that one must accompany his or her planning of evaluation with thoughts of "what can possibly go wrong," but this is the state of affairs, and acceptance of that human condition may be the most important aspect of the state of the art in meeting it. More than just anticipating what can possibly go wrong, the evaluator would do well to remember that Murphy was an optimist and plan accordingly; this, too, is part of that state of the art.

However, there is more than anticipation and preventive action involved; the state of the art includes steps to be taken after problems — anticipated or not — arise. (Some call this "reactive.") Really we are talking about tactics as opposed to strategy. Here we include the arts of diplomacy, of compromise, and perhaps even of benign manipulation. The state of the art has not been changed in a major way over a long period of time. Are we not really talking about the arts of Benjamin Franklin, of Machiavelli, of Disraeli, or Kissinger?

And if that is the case, it seems to me that we need to look to ourselves first. Whether we are part of the problem or indeed just the agent of its solution suggests that we ought to look at ourselves first and "get our own house together." Human relationships can be improved with the development of self-insight along with the development of skills. Crucially important is that first step: how am I contributing to this problem?

All of which reminds me, of course, of a story — this one related to me by the person who experienced something we all have in our work as evaluators. It happened to Mrs. Dunn, who was teaching kindergarten in a suburb of Buffalo — actually at the Harlem Road School in the town of Amherst. She told me that each day she used to line up her charges just before they went home to make sure that their shoes were tied securely. And on one day when she came to the next-to-the-last child, she found his shoes were not tied. Wanting to expedite the whole process, she kneeled down and began to tie his shoes, only to discover that the last little boy, who was awaiting his turn — had apparently walked in a mess of "dog dirt." And suddenly the boy whose shoes she was tying blurted out, "Mrs. Dunn, something smells terrible." Wanting to avoid a problem, Mrs. Dunn said, "Just be patient, Johnny; you'll soon be out of here." But the child persisted, saying, "But Mrs. Dunn, it really smells awful bad." Once again — and hurrying as she did so — Mrs. Dunn said, "Just be a little patient, Johnny." Johnny unfortunately went on, "But Mrs. Dunn, it's gonna make me sick." Exasperated, poor Mrs. Dunn said, "Johnny, I can't help it." Whereupon the child replied, "Oh, 'scuse me, Mrs. Dunn, I didn't know it was you!"

There are two morals to that story. One is the obvious: make sure that you are not part of the problem. The other is that evaluators are going to get blamed for a hell of a lot of things — at least some of which they are innocent of and some of which they cannot control. But that is the nature of our work and learning to be skillful politically can make our professional and technical role an easier one.

11 THE STATE OF THE ART: A SUMMARY STATEMENT

Joseph S. Green

Introduction

This final chapter summarizes the most important contributions made by the faculty of the state-of-the-art Conference on the evaluation of continuing education in the health professions. The first section deals with the purpose, focus, and design of evaluations. Specific quantitative and qualitative techniques are discussed in the second section, followed by a report on the key ideas which relate to politics and methods of implementation, as presented by the Conference speakers.

Purpose, Focus, and Design of Evaluation

The major theme reiterated throughout the Conference dealt with the narrow scope of current continuing-education (CE) evaluations — either experimental research or the determination of whether educational objectives had been met. Several experts agreed that the key evaluation effort should not be solely to *prove* the value of CE per se but rather also to *improve* the quality of individual educational activities. It was suggested that CE must

167

be viewed in the same way as is the medical model: probabilistic, not deterministic. Expanding the focus of CE evaluation was deemed necessary as a way to make evaluations more productive. The design of the evaluations, it was said, should be determined as a result of an analysis of the informational needs of the critical CE decision-makers. Depending upon the purpose(s) of the evaluation, a variety of data-gathering and analysis techniques should be used.

The evaluation design should emerge from the purpose. Two approaches to design present an apparent dichotomy of approaches. One is traditional, positivistic, quantitative while the other is more of a phenomenological, qualitative approach. In reality, it was pointed out, both methods offer a variety of techniques which are of varying utility depending on the purpose of the evaluation and the resources available. The best evaluation design will probably utilize some of each. The role of the evaluator is to get agreement as to the purpose of the evaluation and then to select the most appropriate methods.

A useful conceptualization was presented that suggested three levels of evaluation. The first was for *development* efforts in which the focus is to study the effects of parts of educational programs on participant learners and would include needs assessment and pretesting and posttesting activities. The *demonstration* level would involve trying out entire programs and attempting to ascertain indicators of program effects. The focus at this level would be in determining initial and later status of learners, side effects, and outcomes related to the execution of the entire program. *Research* is the third level and involves true or quasi-experimental design to better understand the actual outcomes of an entire program, while describing cause-and-effect relationships. Most CE evaluation, it was pointed out by the CE evaluator participants, do and should fall into the first two categories. Only when resources warrant it and cause-and-effect relationships are sought should evaluation research be undertaken. If it is, experimental and quasi-experimental methods must be considered as an integral part of any design.

Quantitative and Qualitative Techniques

There were two important themes that surfaced throughout the Conference. The first was that the specific research or evaluation question should not be dictated by a preselected data-analysis procedure. The second was that a variety of quantitative and qualitative techniques ought to be considered, depending on the nature of and purpose for the evaluation effort. The emphasis was on seeking a balance between experimental and naturalistic methods.

The benefits of experimentation using quantifiable data were outlined in detail. Classical experimental design and quasi-experimental designs offer the evaluators methods by which they can build a case for estimating program effects. Random assignment to control and experimental groups, standardized procedures, and validated instruments all assist in the required task of ruling out alternative explanations to discovered effects. A more rigidly controlled evaluation design allows for scheduling of individuals, treatments, observations, and/or measurement to minimize threats to internal validity.

There has been over the past few years an increase in the complexity and multivariate nature of quantitative analysis. The ever-increasing need as a potentially valuable evaluation mechanism in continuing medical education. Finally, what was recommended was the creation of longitudinal data bases for use in performance-monitoring which would in turn open the door for the use of time-series analyses.

Politics and Methods of Implementation

This quantitative, qualitative dichotomy was the center of much of the discussion during the Conference. It was suggested that evaluators have an obligation to their clients to make them aware of their orientation. In addition, more needs to be done to make funding agencies more aware of the value of something other than a "scientific" approach to data-gathering and analysis.

Most experts agreed that there has been an increase in attention paid to reporting of results. CE evaluators, it was cautioned, need to be careful and not get into the untenable situation of trying to demonstrate the worth of programs. If they are not successful in "sharing" the worth of their bosses' program, they might lose their jobs.

Four sources of political problems were discussed: (1) monitoring evaluation standards; (2) applying evaluation principles; (3) getting key people to reach necessary agreements; and (4) obtaining compliance among participants. It was pointed out that potential conflicts usually arise over different values held by sponsors, evaluators, and program directors. More evaluations have been foiled due to lack of interpersonal skills on the part of the evaluator than lack of technical skills. In order to prevent possible problems, several suggestions were put forth: anticipate problems prior to finalizing the design; establish standard operating procedures; describe grievance procedures if conflicts arise; use mediation procedures to resolve differences among key audiences. After the evaluation was under way, other suggestions included: using diplomacy; compromising; using arbitration; surrendering.

Suggestions for the Future

In order to move ahead, the field of evaluation of continuing education in the health professions, five suggestions are put forth by the editors. First, a National Continuing Education Evaluation Coordinating Council should be established to monitor evaluation studies. Second, a major task of this group would be to provide leadership to the field by establishing a set of priorities for evaluation-research questions. The third suggestion is to make this priority list available to all involved in CE evaluation in the health professions to guide them in their efforts. Fourth, a yearly research and evaluation conference is suggested as a method of sharing results, reexamining priorities, and providing awards for the best efforts of the year. Finally, training should be made available to all evaluators of continuing education in the specifics of both quantitative and qualitative methodologies.

Index

Name Index